DON'T JUST LIE THERE...

Michael van Straten's Guide to Good Sleep

with illustrations by
Marie-Hélène Jeeves

TO MY FATHER, LOUIS VAN STRATEN
whom I have never ever known to have a sleepless night,
who can sleep anywhere at any time,
and who has snored his way obliviously through 82 years.

First published 1990 in Great Britain by
Kyle Cathie Limited
3 Vincent Square London SW1P 2LX

The amount of sleep that the average person needs always seems to be about five minutes more than they get. There is an epidemic of 'sleep obsession' spreading throughout the western world. Too much, too little, too disturbed, too deep, too light, too dream-free, too dream-laden, too much or too little of everything and never just right.

Disruption of sleep patterns is not a disease, merely a symptom of some underlying cause, and the commonest of all the sleep disturbances is insomnia. Insomnia is most emphatically not a disease: all the more surprising then that it is so often treated with powerful and frequently habituating, if not always addictive, drugs.

To limp through life on a crutch of sleeping pills or tranquillisers as the sole means of ensuring what is considered to be 'a good night's sleep', is a needless sentence which is so often handed down as a matter of expediency by the doctor or is self-inflicted by the patient who demands a magic pill as the easiest way of solving the problem.

Why then, as an alternative practitioner, am I moved to write this book? After 25 years in practice and more than ten years as the Alternative Medicine Man on London's LBC radio station, I rank insomnia high in the Top Ten list of ailments for which people seek my advice. Everyone has occasional sleepless nights, although sleepless rarely means totally sleepless. Most people who claim to have not slept a wink have usually managed three or four hours, if not more. Sadly, the memories of the hours spent tossing and turning are far more powerful.

There are many possible causes of insomnia. Which of us doesn't recognise the anxiety of a difficult day ahead, interview, exam, wedding, catching a plane, or for that matter any emotional situation, whether happy or sad? Who hasn't tossed and turned while rehashing every word of a row at work, with a relative or partner? How many of the bereaved lie awake at night regretting things said or unsaid, done or not done? These and all the other conceivable emotional situations are almost certainly the most common triggers of disturbed sleep.

Any physical illness which causes pain will disturb your sleep. A cold, a cough, the flu, bronchitis, asthma, hay fever, irritating skin conditions, a boil on the bottom, an aching tooth, backache, headache, urinary problems, or even a good old-fashioned bout of the 'runs', will certainly separate you from your beauty sleep.

Snoring is a two-edged sword. Not only does it obviously disturb the non-snoring partner, but it frequently has serious effects on the snorer himself – I deliberately say himself as it is most often the male of the species who excels in this department! The snorer is likely to have very disturbed sleep patterns of which he is unaware, but the results of which can seriously interfere with health.

One of the most distressing causes of insomnia is the non-sleeping child. No-one who has never had one of these car possibly imagine the nightmare of years of wakefulness and sleep deprivation. This never seems to have any effect on the child, who will wake the next morning, having seemingly slept for about seven and a half minutes in the past 12 hours, full of energy and as bright as a button. Meanwhile, the bleary parents look forward to another day of fighting against overwhelming fatigue with the prospect of a repeat performance the following night.

Dieting, sex, modern technology, central heating, noisy neighbours and the things we eat and drink all have a part to play in our sleep. Shift work, jet lag, insufficient leisure, too little exercise and, above all, not knowing how to relax can interfere with the most important factor affecting our sleep: habitual patterns which we are programmed to follow.

The phenomenal growth in all aspects of complementary medicine has come about because the general public, in growing numbers, no longer wishes just to be prescribed a pill. Modern patients want to be involved in their own treatment, want to participate, want to be informed and want to have some measure of control. It would be foolish to deny the huge benefits of modern medicine. Advances in surgery and drug therapy have brought untold relief, but the tide is turning. The 'pill for every ill' approach no longer satisfies many patients or practitioners and treating the person rather than the symptom is the order of the day. Insomnia is a prime case for the holistic approach and this is what you will find in this book.

The real importance of insomnia is often less than the perception of it. Worrying about the number of hours of sleep or the quality of sleep which you get in any one night, or indeed as a general rule, is bound to create more problems than your actual sleeping habits. Of course sleep is important, but most of us need less than we imagine and can survive on far less than that. None of this matters, though, if you believe that your particular sleeping problem is having an adverse effect on your health and performance. This book is written just for you. You may not like all the answers, you may not find the magic wand which somebody else can wave on your behalf. You will find lots of practical help, simple tips, safe remedies, a little light relief and some good bedtime reading.

The majority of problems fall into one of two categories: an inability to get to sleep, or problems with staying asleep. In the first situation, the likely causes are stress, tension and anxiety; caffeine, alcohol or stimulant drugs; emotional problems; change of surroundings or noise; any form of pain; worries about the effects of lack of sleep.

Waking after only a few hours' sleep, or a long time before you need to get up, may be linked to drugs or alcohol; pain; depression; change of surroundings; restless leg syndrome (involuntary twitching of the leg muscles); breathing difficulties, most often related to snoring (sleep apnoea); low blood sugar due to not eating enough of the right food at the right time.

As you can see, some of these factors are interchangeable, and it isn't always possible to make clear-cut divisions between the two problems. There are some diseases and some prescribed drugs which may interfere with your sleep patterns, but by far the most common cause of all sleep disorders is a psychological problem, which may or may not have its roots in physical disease. Back pain, for example, will keep you awake, but if it takes weeks or even months to get better, your pattern of sleep will have been disrupted. The anxiety over the pain and that caused by loss of sleep, loss of income and possible loss of work, is certain to produce a psychological overlay. This becomes an established pattern of behaviour and will remain imprinted in the subconscious long after the original back condition has been resolved. Whatever the cause, insomnia is a miserable and wretched condition. Long term, eradication of the causes is the only possible solution, but the difficult part is identifying them. If it were easy, there would be no insomniacs, and there would surely be no need for this book. What makes the situation so much harder is the fact that all insomniacs have the roots of their problem in their own life and background. For this reason, there is no simple answer, no miracle cure, no instant relief. There may be 20 possible reasons for your personal situation. There may be 40 possible remedies. The answer which will solve your insomnia may be a combination of any two, 22, or all 40. It's a bit like doing the pools, and only you can work out your own personal perm.

To be an ex-insomniac you've got to do it yourself: no-one else can do it to you. So – DON'T JUST LIE THERE . . .

1

2 – 4 – 6 – 8 – . . .
HOW MANY HOURS DO WE NEED AND OTHER MYTHS

'Early to bed and early to rise makes a man healthy, wealthy and wise.'

Proverb

'One hour's sleep before midnight is worth two after.'

Proverb

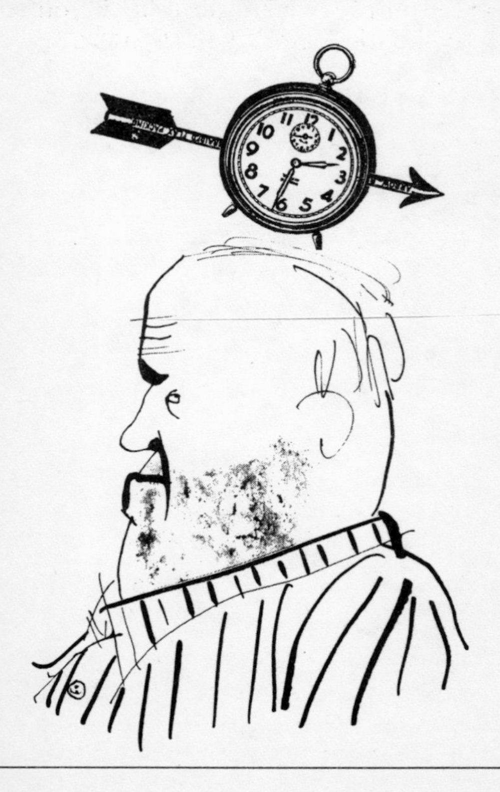

The whole question of how much sleep we need and when we need it is a minefield of myth and folklore. There are those who pride themselves on never getting more than five hours a night, and others who obsessively demand a full nine hours in the belief that five minutes less will ruin their lives.

The truth is probably somewhere between the two, although nobody knows for sure. One certain thing is that the odd disturbed night or the occasional patch of insomnia does no harm. What does the damage is the anxiety and stress which some people suffer as a result of their own perception of the harm that can be caused by lack of sleep. Leaving aside sleep disorders caused by actual disease, most other sleep problems are brought upon the sufferers themselves or inflicted on them by friends, relatives or doctors who insist on perpetuating the myth that we need eight hours' sleep each and every night.

There is a great deal of mystery and a slowly growing body of fact about sleep, and if you are seriously determined to unravel the cause of your insomnia, or to understand your sleeping patterns and needs sufficiently to realise that you do not suffer from insomnia, the first step is to separate the fact from the fiction, the myth from the reality, and the old wives' tale from practical common sense.

Many years ago I had the privilege of knowing one of the great paediatricians, Dr David Morris. He was a man of infinite patience with babies and children, limitless common sense and immense professional ability. His tolerance did not always extend to his patients' parents and when asked repeatedly by one young mother for help with a very wakeful baby, he finally wrote out a prescription for a sedative. The mother was horrified and exclaimed that she wasn't going to give that sort of drug to her baby.

Not without a hint of sarcasm, Dr Morris replied that if she was so concerned with her baby's wakefulness, she and her husband could take it in turns to take the medicine; that way at least 'You'll get your eight hours' beauty sleep every other night.'

This doctor was wise enough to know that sleep is a matter of different strokes for different folks, and babies are no exception. It may be that your optimum sleeping pattern has been disturbed and you are suffering as a consequence. It may also be that the sleeping pattern which your body wants to adopt differs from that which you think is best for your health. Either way, knowledge and understanding will overcome the problem.

Forget the old wives' tales, especially the sheep. Put aside all your preconceived ideas about what sleep is, how much you need, when you need it, and where you should have it. You are about to embark on a journey across the Styx to a land of golden slumbers. This is a voyage of discovery and reality, of peace and dreams, and above all of self-awareness. I hope you will find the solution to your problems somewhere in the following pages, but if all else fails, turn on the light and start the next chapter – that's bound to work.

Sleep and Civilisation

Way back during our evolutionary process we were cold-blooded water creatures, and as we evolved, so our bodily functions changed, including the way in which we sleep. Our sleeping time falls into two phases. The predominant phase consists of periods of orthodox or non-rapid eye movements (NREM sleep). These are interspersed with short periods of unorthodox or paradoxical sleep during which there are rapid eye movements (REM sleep), and it is possibly these periods which are left over from our aquatic ancestors. From the time of the cavemen through till the beginning of the 19th century, our sleep patterns hardly changed. They were governed by the seasons, the sun and the moon. Periods of sleep were decreed by cold and dark, and periods of wakeful activity by sun and the demands of hunting, gathering or harvesting food.

The Industrial Revolution brought sweeping changes: a dramatic shift of the population from country to city; power for heating and lighting; the noise of thousands of families living in confined areas and in close proximity to factories where shiftwork became the established norm.

No longer was it early to bed and early to rise with the going down and coming up of the sun. For the first time in man's history the patterns of sleep were not in tune with the rhythms of nature. And that's when all the trouble started. Working hours which don't fit with our inborn biological time clock, together with social pressures which produce irregular sleeping patterns and more specific problems like jet lag, all conspire to disrupt the regularity of our sleep and so to interfere with the amount we get, and its quality.

Most of us spend a third of our lives sleeping; we have special rooms for it, special clothes for it and special furniture to do it in, and yet exactly what is sleep? The truth is that we don't know and despite the technology of the electroencephalogram and the growing amount of research done in sleep laboratories, the precise nature of sleep remains a mystery.

To help you understand more about your own problem, let's look more closely at some of the things we do know.

There are a number of factors which singly or in combination can be the trigger which sends us to sleep. When any individual reaches the time of day when they would normally expect to go to sleep, the approximate hour to which they have become conditioned, they will feel sleepy. Excessive warmth, a full stomach, sex, boredom will all also contribute to us feeling sleepy.

The circadian rhythm which governs the way our bodies work during the 24 hour day is something which we have in common with all other living creatures, and plants, too, for that matter. If you keep a simple temperature chart for three or four days and fill it in every couple of hours, you will see that your body temperature is highest in the middle of the day and lowest in the middle of the night. Even shift-workers, who reverse the normal pattern, will find that their temperature is lowest in the middle of the night, even though they are awake and working. No matter how hard you try, you can't fool this natural rhythm. Ask anyone who has a night time job and they will tell you that no matter how well they have slept during the day, when it gets to three o'clock in the morning it's a struggle to keep awake, concentrate and perform efficiently. As soon as dawn breaks, they perk up and by the time they get home at eight or nine in the morning, when by all logical reasoning they should feel exhausted, many people find it difficult to go to sleep. Their circadian rhythms tell their bodies that this is daytime, a time for being up and doing, not for sleeping.

Within our 24 hour biological clock we have another rhythm, the ultradian rhythm, and this follows a cycle of around 100 minutes. Although the ultradian cycle is with us throughout the 24 hours, its effects are most apparent when we sleep (though mainly to observers, not sleepers). It is possible to notice the effects of this secondary cycle during enforced periods of inactivity – during long plane journeys, for instance, or if you are bedbound through some injury like a broken leg which doesn't make you ill. There is an obvious tendency for behaviour patterns to change roughly every 100 minutes. Restlessness, drowsiness, hunger, laziness, these sorts of feelings are part of the clock within the clock. Imagine a 24 hour clock with an hour hand that makes a complete circle once in each 24 hours and a sweep hand which makes a complete circle once in every 100 minutes. This gives you an idea of how the two cycles come together. When the sleep hour arrives at the same time as a sleepy period in the 100 minute cycle, then sleep will come easily.

But this should happen at the same time each day, so why do people have problems? The answer is that often we don't allow ourselves to go to sleep when our bodies are primed to do it.

One of the few old wives' tales about sleep which has more than a grain of truth in it is the one that says sleep is essential for growing children. Whilst there is no evidence that children who sleep less are smaller, or that children who sleep a great deal are bigger, it is a fact that hormones play a large part in sleep and that growth hormone particularly is produced during sleep and in greater abundance during deep orthodox sleep. For this reason much of the body's repair work is done whilst we dream the night away. The skin is revitalised by the growth of new cells and more of them are produced during sleep. It doesn't take many sleepless nights for the skin to show visible effects. In the brain and the eyes protein is replaced faster whilst you sleep. Sleep is a time of building up whilst waking is a time of breaking down. This happens because of a different set of hormones, those in more abundant supply at times of activity.

Adrenalin circulates throughout the body whenever we are awake and active, though in quite small quantities. This is the hormone that activates our fright, fight or flight response to external stimuli. It is one of the most primitive of mechanisms and certainly one that has done the most to keep *homo sapiens* going through the ages. The body's instant response to a threatening situation is to release vast quantities of adrenalin into the bloodstream. This increases the blood pressure, the heart rate and the speed at which you breathe, carrying more oxygen to the muscles together with the nutrients they need for sustained activity, and thus preparing you to fight or run away. The old stories of the man chased by a bull leaping a five-barred gate without hesitation are true, and it's all down to adrenalin.

The other important group of hormones produced while we are awake are the corticosteroids, which work hand in hand with adrenalin. They are released into the bloodstream just before you wake and it's these which make you leap out of bed ready and willing to face another day – that is, of course, if you go to bed and get up regularly at the same time.

Both of these 'activity' hormones interfere with the work of growth hormones. When you are busy getting on with life during the daytime your body can't spare the energy required for growing, repairing and restoring and these hormones make sure that this doesn't happen. The reverse occurs at night-time: the activity hormones drop to a very low level, so enabling the growth hormone to stimulate the body to get on with the job of repair. An interesting benefit of understanding this pattern has been used in the treatment of children who are deficient in human growth hormone. Expert endocrinologists at child growth clinics have found that giving children their dose of growth hormones at night-time is more effective than administering the medicine during the day.

This also highlights one of the most important factors causing poor quality sleep. How often have you woken in the morning knowing that you have really slept for a good number of hours and yet struggled to drag yourself awake and felt down, lethargic and generally one degree under for the rest of the day? This happens when your production of the daytime and night-time hormones gets out of kilter. Ideally you should have the most growth hormone and the least adrenalin during the night, and the most adrenalin and the least growth hormone during the day. As a result of an irregular lifestyle – commonly in people who work split shifts or night shifts, who frequently paint the town till the small hours, and, most of all, insomniacs – this hormone pattern is disturbed. Instead you may end up not producing enough growth hormone when you are awake all night; when you sleep during the day you might produce the hormone, but its effect will be nullified by the high levels of adrenalin. The net result is that your body misses out on its routine maintenance and you feel jaded.

There is no treatment for your fighting hormones. The only solution is to try to regulate your sleep patterns and we shall see how to do that in Chapter 3. But now for more about sleep itself.

Some of the early observers of sleep noticed that at certain times babies appeared to move their eyes rapidly whilst they were obviously still sleeping. This seemed to happen at frequent intervals throughout their sleeping periods and be interspersed with longer times during which they didn't move their eyes. It was originally assumed that the eye movements were a result of dreams.

It was not until the early 1950s that researchers in Chicago made use of the electroencephalogram to investigate brain-waves and sleep. These scientists, too, observed that there were times during sleep in which the sleeper's eyes made rapid movements, and it was at this time that Aserinsky and Kleitman started waking up their subjects during these periods of rapid eye movement, which they found in everyone, and were surprised to find that most people woken at this point in their sleep were able to describe their dreams. This was the start of serious sleep research and enabled scientists to build up a picture of how we go to sleep and what happens in the brain when we do.

When you turn off the TV at the end of the movie and go to bed your brain waves show a normal waking pattern. As you relax you drift into a period of half sleep during which the rest of the world fades into the distance, your muscles relax and the electrical activity in your brain settles to a steady rhythm of alpha waves. If, at this point, the phone rings or the baby cries, the alpha rhythm stops, adrenalin is produced and you are once again wide awake. If all goes well, the electrical activity slows even more and you move into Stage 1 sleep. If you are serious about going to sleep, and not just dozing in the armchair, you progress to Stage 2 sleep with even slower brain waves. These get larger and slower still in Stage 3 and even slower in Stage 4. In all these stages there are no eye movements and it becomes progressively more difficult to arouse the sleeper as the stages progress. You are less likely to remember dreams during these stages and if you do, they will probably be mundane and boring. All four stages make up orthodox or NREM sleep.

Between each of these stages is a short period of sleep during which rapid eye movements are present. These stages are the unorthodox, paradoxical sleep or REM. It's usual for approximately 80% of sleep to be orthodox and 20% to be paradoxical, and the brain waves found during paradoxical sleep are smaller and quicker than those in deep sleep. It's hard to say whether either of these two types of sleep is more important than the other, but they are certainly very different. Whilst sleep is deeper in orthodox, in paradoxical, muscles are far more relaxed, sometimes to the point of paralysis.

Mental activity carries on during both forms of sleep, but there are differences. Experimental subjects woken from orthodox sleep describe what they have been 'thinking' as opposed to the vivid dream descriptions of those woken during paradoxical sleep. The divisions between these two events are very sharp and if waking from paradoxical sleep is delayed by just a few minutes so that the subject is into the start of the next orthodox sleep cycle, the memory of dreams is much less clear. Sleep-walking and night terrors (see page 63) tend to happen during the early stages of orthodox sleep and they are never remembered the following morning. There is generally very little that happens during sleep which is remembered on waking, and the concept of 'sleep learning' – using tape recorders playing while you sleep to learn a language, for example – is a waste of time. The only thing you are likely to remember is what you heard before you fell asleep. You can't learn without concentrating and paying attention, neither of which is possible while you sleep.

Nevertheless, sleep is vital for the proper functioning of

your memory and there are suggestions that paradoxical sleep is the time during which the thoughts and activities of the day are programmed into the memory bank of the brain's computer. There are other differences between the two types of sleep. For instance if volunteers are deprived of Stage 4 sleep they tend to be very tired and apathetic the next day. If, on the other hand, you stop them having paradoxical sleep, then the memory is affected, together with the ability to acquire skills. It's also been found that if a subject is deprived of paradoxical sleep for two or three nights and then allowed to sleep normally, the periods of paradoxical sleep will be lengthened to make up for those lost in the previous nights. Sleeping pills and tranquillisers can have an adverse effect on the relative proportions of orthodox and paradoxical sleep, and these drugs are best avoided wherever possible (see Chapter 5).

All the current research would seem to point to the fact that both quantity and quality of sleep are important, though faced with the choice of one or the other, quality would certainly win. Quality means the right relationship between growth hormones and activity hormones, and the establishment of as regular a pattern of sleeping as is consistent with each individual's lifestyle and the demands of their job and social life.

As for the amount of sleep required, this is without doubt the classic 'how long is a piece of string' question. There is a feeling that short sleepers are the doers of this world and the long sleepers the dullards, but this does not strictly speaking appear to be true. What evidence there is suggests that short sleepers do indeed tend to be thrusting, decisive people – politicians, the heads of big corporations, eminent scientists and doctors. Long sleepers, on the other hand, are more creative, more eccentric, and frequently greater individualists at an intellectual level.

All one can say for certain is that 'enough' sleep is what is enough for you as an individual, regardless of what the norm is generally accepted to be. If you suffer long-term deprivation in the amount of sleep you need, the consequences are serious. Very few people cope successfully with less than four to five hours' sleep on a regular basis. If they get that sleep in one uninterrupted segment they will certainly be better off than the person who has ten hours constantly interrupted by outside factors or their own intrinsic sleep problems. Stories of people who 'never' sleep are not to be believed. Sleep deprivation makes people sleepy and it is extremely hard to stop someone who has not slept for three consecutive nights from falling asleep. Anyone would be badly affected in this situation. Their concentration would be minimal, their decision-making abilities impaired, their attention span severely limited. They would possibly have hallucinations and would certainly drift off into repeated 'micro sleeps', sometimes in mid-conversation or even with their spoon halfway to their mouth.

One of the most disturbing myths about sleep is that which warns of the danger of madness if you do not have enough paradoxical sleep and consequently do not dream enough. This story grew out of a very flawed study in which the subjects were told to expect some psychological disturbances but also had available to them the services of an on-call psychiatrist in case of any crisis. Needless to say, the volunteers showed considerable signs of mental disturbance. Reports of this study filled the media for months and the idea of dream deprivation and madness became firmly established in the public mind. When the same researchers repeated the study more carefully, none of the volunteers suffered psychiatric problems, just the normal results of sleep deprivation. But the damage haa already been done. The popular press weren't interested. 'Lack of dreams causes madness' is a great headline. 'Lack of dreams doesn't cause madness after all' is not.

How much is normal?

There have been many experimental attempts to establish what is the normal amount of sleep that we require. To date there is no definitive answer, save that as we've already seen individual requirements vary from person to person, but we do know what average sleeping habits are in a large cross-section of the population. Some 66% of people sleep for anything between six and a half and eight and a half hours each night on a regular basis. Around 16% sleep for more than eight and a half hours each night, and 18% for under six and a half hours. This would seem to be a reasonable estimation of what most people do most of the time. However, this does not mean that variations beyond these figures make you 'abnormal'. There is a comparatively small percentage of the population, which nevertheless represents a very substantial number of people, who consistently sleep for less than five hours each night. These so-called short sleepers have the normal ultradian rhythm of orthodox and paradoxical sleep in approximately 100 minute cycles. What is unusual about them is that they seem to do without the stages of light sleep and go straight from waking into deep sleep which, as we've already seen, is the time when the smallest quantity of activity hormones and the largest amount of growth hormone are circulating in the bloodstream.

This pattern seems to be eminently suitable to those who have it; they suffer no harmful side effects, and frequently turn out to be the active 'doers' in our society. So it would be quite wrong to describe these people as abnormal sleepers. It's also important to realise that normal sleeping patterns do change with age. New-born babies differ hugely from three-year-old toddlers, and the octogenarian will have completely different sleeping habits from those of an 18-year-old. Leaving aside any external factors which might occasionally alter sleeping patterns, the 18-year-old will have far fewer interruptions during a night's sleep than a 40-year-old, who will in turn have less interrupted sleep than a 70-year-old, who will have better sleep than a 90-year-old. For some reason older men appear to suffer more sleep interruptions than older women.

The amount of paradoxical sleep in any night does not vary much with age; what does change is the proportion of time spent in deep sleep. A 75-year-old will enjoy just as much paradoxical sleep as an 18-year-old, but somewhat less than half the amount of Stage 3 and 4 deep sleep. This is why many older people find it necessary, and often unavoidable, to doze during the daytime, as they are frequently deprived of the restorative effect of Stage 4 sleep.

The effects of loss of sleep

Apart from the obvious result of making you feel tired, sleep loss can have more far-reaching effects. Many studies have been done both on people totally deprived of sleep for periods of two or three nights, on volunteers whose total sleep has been reduced gradually over a period of time, and on subjects whose sleep has been interrupted so as to deprive them of a variety of stages of sleep.

Gradual reduction of sleep in a group of volunteers produced an interesting result. A group of subjects whose normal sleeping time was around seven hours a night had this gradually reduced to five hours. This seemed to have very little effect on their ability to perform physical tasks or on their mental agility, but they all felt extremely tired and found that five hours' sleep was the absolute minimum on which they could manage.

A lot of attention has been focused on junior hospital doctors and their excessively long working hours. Fears have been expressed that the lack of sleep which these young professionals have to suffer could have serious implications for their patients. These fears are nothing new. As long ago as 1971 and 1975 studies on young doctors in both England and America showed that there were indeed alarming problems posed by the demands placed on them. The majority were themselves concerned about their loss of efficiency, and although some people coped better than others when deprived of sleep, the overall results indicated a greater likelihood of mistakes, reduction in memory capability which led to difficulties in interpreting information from patients, short-temperedness, irritability and rudeness to both patients and nursing staff – behaviour about which they subsequently felt guilty and ashamed.

One of the key factors involved in sleep loss seems to be frequent lapses in memory and concentration. The ability to perform single specific tasks doesn't appear to be worse after a sleepless night. In fact, the reaction time needed to respond to simple tests like pressing a button to switch off a flashing light can be just as quick in some subjects as that required after a good night's sleep. But faced with repetitive reaction-time tests, or tasks which involve continuous concentration and which are not in themselves in any way exciting or stimulating, performance shows a rapid decline.

The ability to make reasoned, calculated decisions is also diminished, and this could have serious consequences for the international businessman when faced with jet lag and varying time zones. Most large companies now appreciate the significance of meddling with the biological time clock, and few employers would expect, or even allow, their executives to get straight off a plane and go to an important business meeting. I am always horrified by chairmen, managing directors, chief executives and very senior professionals like lawyers, accountants or financiers who believe that they are the exceptions to the rule. The rules which they make for their more junior colleagues don't seem to apply to them. They have some misguided macho image which compels them to believe that they are unaffected by boring factors like jet lag or sleep loss. I see patients who catch the morning flight to New York, go straight to a business lunch, sit in meetings all the afternoon, have a night on the town with their colleagues, go to bed, don't sleep, get up, catch the morning flight to Los Angeles, do it all again, catch the overnight flight to London, and go straight to the office. Often they repeat this performance every week or so and sometimes the schedule is even more punishing. The extraordinary thing is that these highly intelligent captains of industry behave in such an irresponsible way often to the detriment of their companies and their shareholders. What's more, when they have their first heart attack, certainly sooner rather than later, their universal cry is, 'What have I done to deserve this?'

Most western countries have strict controls over the number of hours which people in certain occupations are allowed to work without a rest period. Bus, coach and lorry drivers, airline pilots, train and underground drivers all come within some form of legal constraint. Unfortunately there are no regulations which govern the working hours of doctors, lawyers, businessmen or, most importantly, mothers. It's hardly surprising that mistakes happen, that bad decisions are made, or that mothers find themselves at the end of their tethers and often fearful of inflicting violence on their children.

As you will discover throughout this book, there are many causes of poor sleep and lack of sleep, and equally there are many ways in which you can help to improve both quality and quantity of this precious ingredient of good health. A lot of sleep problems involve our own inbuilt biological clock and the ways in which we ignore it, tamper with it or try to impose our social demands on to it. This clock does not like change and will show its disapproval by making you feel sleepy or awake at inconvenient times. With care it is possible to adjust your time clock and your lifestyle so that the two are more compatible.

Nobody knows for certain where these clocks come from or how they survive. Are they just the body's response to the natural rhythms of day and night, or are they some internal mechanism programmed into our genetic structure? And what about the rhythms within the rhythm? In laboratory studies it is not difficult to isolate animals, plants or tissue cultures from the external effects of heat and light, and even in these conditions there appears to be a regular pattern to their activities. There don't seem to be exceptions – even a turnip is able to demonstrate cyclical patterns of activity!

Changes in magnetic field strength and even variations in gravitational pull coinciding with phases of the moon are known to have an effect on many organisms, and it is virtually impossible to screen experimental subjects from these. Folklore and mythology abound with stories of the moon's cycle affecting human behaviour and a growing number of people believe that magnetic fields such as those generated by overhead cables, by domestic power circuits and even by sunspots, do have a powerful effect on the human body and mind. For centuries there have been old wives' tales about which way one should sleep in relation to the earth's magnetic field, and although this may seem like hocus pocus, serious scientific research continues into the effects that magnetism has on the human biological clock. There are dowsers who, as well as finding water with their famous forked sticks, will also tell you in which direction to place your bed in your house. There are experts on ley lines who will even tell you where to build your house and there are companies manufacturing devices which will isolate your bedroom from the electrical circuits to avoid creating magnetic loops which supposedly interfere with your sleep and health.

Even the weather can affect the quantity and quality of your sleep. High humidity, violent storms with their accompanying very low pressure, the hot winds that blow across Europe from the deserts can all have adverse effects. Ionised air is reputed to encourage good sleep and these days you no longer have to go to the seaside or the famous spas to get your dose of ozone. You can buy a small electronic ioniser which will run in your bedroom with, to my knowledge, extremely beneficial effects on some people's sleep.

Whatever the cause of your problem, you will find some answers in the following chapters. In many respects quality of sleep is more important than quantity, and the key to arriving at a better balance between the two, of changing your sleeping habits (even if they are the habits of a lifetime) and of banishing the nightmare of insomnia depends on overcoming disorder and creating order in the way you approach your individual need for sleep.

2

GOOD HABITS, BAD HABITS

'I haven't been to sleep for over a year. That's why I go to bed early. One needs more rest if one doesn't sleep.'

Evelyn Waugh

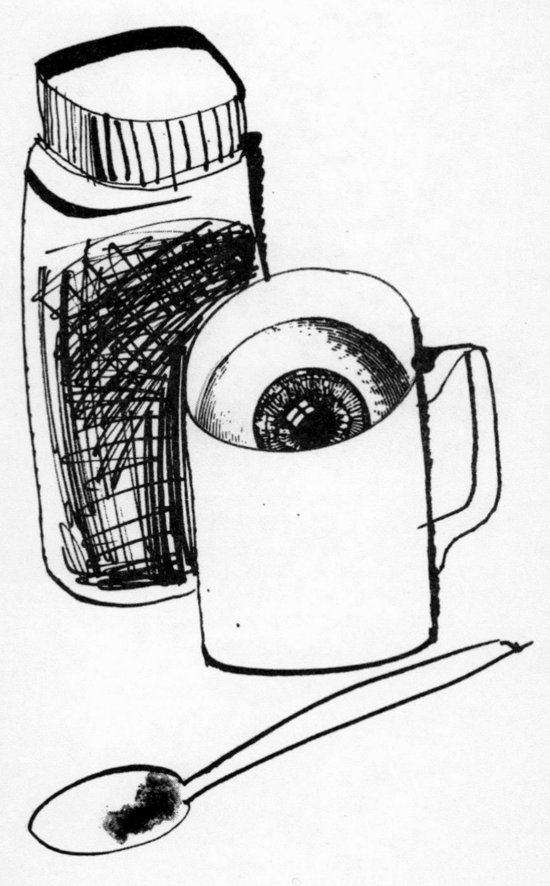

We are all creatures of habit. Like it or not, our day-to-day lives follow predictable patterns. Even the most disorganised people have a pattern to their chaos. Many of our activities are governed by learned responses which are imprinted in our subconscious. In this respect we are no different from Pavlov's dogs. By using a mixture of food and bells he was able to train his dogs to salivate at the sound of the bell before they even saw or smelled the food, and his experiments led to our understanding of the 'conditioned reflex'.

Within our bodily system there are many built-in reflexes over which we have little or no control: the knee jerk and the blinking eye are obvious examples. Thanks to Pavlov we now know that we can develop other reflex patterns of behaviour, laid down by circumstances which condition us to produce identical responses in given situations. With enough repetition these responses become an inherent part of our lifestyle. We develop habits, good and bad.

Nowhere are these habits more important than in relation to the question of sleep, or lack of it. As we have seen already, good sleep is dependent on fitting in with the predetermined rhythms of our bodily sleep cycle, and the 24 hour variations in body temperature. A major problem facing habitual insomniacs is the pattern into which they fall in a vain attempt to come to terms with their problems. They acquire habits of wakefulness when they should be sleeping, and sleepiness when they should be awake.

Lifestyle habits play a key role in determining sleep patterns, as do those imposed by occupational demands, family commitments and the environment in which we live. There are some habits which, for practical reasons, it is not possible to change. But unless it is an essential part of the working life, there is no acquired habit which cannot be changed with sufficient commitment and practice. Learning new habits is not difficult – you can teach any old dog new tricks. The most difficult part is forgetting the old habits. Those which are deeply ingrained and have become reflex patterns built into the microcircuitry of our subconscious.

To illustrate how hard it can be to eradicate some of these acquired reflexes totally, think of the problems of changing your car after a year or so of familiarity. For the first few weeks you instinctively move the right-hand lever on the steering column to work the indicators, and in fact you turn on the windscreen wipers. In your old car it was the left-hand lever for the wipers and the right for the indicators. It doesn't take long to get used to the new layout, and you are soon using the right switch for the right purpose without even thinking about it.

Until, that is, an emergency arises. You have to act instantly – no time to think, no time to reason, just a reflex action – what do you do? You turn on the windscreen wipers instead of the indicators. And this can happen months after you acquired the new vehicle. That's how hard it is to forget old habits.

The world is full of infuriating people who spend a lifetime breaking all the rules that we are supposed to follow in order to ensure a sound night's sleep, and yet never seem to have a problem. They can drink gallons of coffee, eat seven-course dinners late at night, fly across time zones, never exercise, watch horror movies till three in the morning, have rows with their partners just after going to bed, and, in spite of all, the minute their head hits the pillow they're out like a light. Any one of these things can spell disaster for the difficult sleeper, yet 'they' seem to get away with all of them and still come up bright-eyed and bushy-tailed in time for breakfast. There's no justice.

For most people, though there are basic rules covering bad habits to avoid or change and good habits that are worth acquiring. The times at which you get up and go to bed, the amount of physical exercise you take, the way you respond to emotionally difficult situations, the success or otherwise of your personal relationships, what you wear or don't wear in bed, the type of bed you sleep in, the condition of your bedroom; all these will affect you to a greater or lesser extent. Your success in establishing new and better paths to peaceful nights will depend on how much change you can make in all these variables. It's just like balancing an equation and if you can solve the puzzle you will succeed. Only a fool would suggest that there is an infallible solution to insomnia. There are lots of solutions just as there are lots of insomniacs. The trick is to work out the best combination of solutions for any given individual, and you are the only person who can solve your specific sleep equation.

Eating, drinking, not eating, not drinking, alcohol, caffeine, exercise, too much exercise, emotional problems, too much sex, not enough sex, excitement, ritual, the type of bed, or even the position of your bed, can all be positive or negative influences on the way you sleep. Some insomniacs have difficulty getting to sleep, others nod off quite peacefully but can't stay asleep and wake in the small hours. Just how the various habits which we adopt affect the patterns of our sleep is often a mystery, but it is certainly a fact that all these things can exert a powerful influence.

Getting out of the bad habits only takes a little willpower, and getting into the good ones a little practice. Make a list of the good and bad ones that you have, then keep a diary for two or three weeks and see how successful you can be at implementing your new regime for better sleep. Don't forget to include in your list everything you eat and drink each day during this period. You may be amazed and horrified by the amount of caffeine and alcohol you consume, both of which will adversely affect your sleep patterns. When and how much you eat are both important, as is your pattern of work and social activities, especially during the evening.

Food

Different types of food and their effects on sleep are the manna of myth and folklore. Not surprisingly, there is more than a grain of truth in many of the old wives' tales and any of them may be keeping you awake, or could help to get you off to sleep.

When and what you eat is the first consideration. Going to bed hungry is a surefire recipe for a disturbed night. Not only do the gnawing pains in your empty stomach, and the rumblings that it produces, inevitably wake you up at three in the morning, but the low level of sugar in the blood circulating to your brain is also an important factor.

The modern obsession with dieting and weight loss is, I am quite sure, just one more ingredient in the recipe for the growing number of insomniacs (around 20 million people in the UK are likely to have some sleep problems during their lives). Obesity certainly brings its own problems to the bedroom, more of that later. But the habitual dieter runs the risk of falling into the trap of a vicious circle. When the dieting becomes extreme and the spectre of anorexia looms on the horizon, this risk becomes even greater. Anyone desperately sticking to a very low calorie diet is going to lack energy. They will almost certainly have a substandard level of nutrition and will be permanently hungry. This will interfere with sleep and lead to phsyical and mental exhaustion. The inevitable consequence is depression, and depression will lead to even worse sleep and even worse eating habits.

If you are determined to lose weight or indeed, if you need to lose weight, do it sensibly. Extreme diets always lead to disaster, mainly because no one can stick to them for long. In my practice I have spent 25 years watching people making themselves thoroughly miserable with the latest diet fad, losing a stone in ten days, and putting on a stone and a half in the following week. This pattern is not good for your health and will certainly disrupt your normal sleeping habits and leave you dissatisfied, convinced that you are a failure and, just to add insult to injury, an insomniac. Most dieters, and indeed the majority of doctors, are still under the impression that carbohydrates are bad news for would-be thinnies. This is far from the truth, since the complex carbohydrates – wholemeal bread, wholegrain cereals, brown rice, pasta, lentils and all the pulses – are an excellent source of nutrients, a minimal source of fats and essential for good sleep. There seems to be a link between high carbohydrate foods and the body's production of the chemical serotonin, which plays an important part in our sleep mechanism (see page 76). So apart from sending you to bed hungry, which will inevitably give you sleepless nights, the low calorie and very low calorie diets interfere with the physiology of sleep.

The simplest way to lose weight is to cut out all the visible fats, and to avoid the invisible fats: these are the ones hidden in biscuits, cakes, sausages, salamis, meat pies, bolognese sauce, chocolates, crisps and many prefabricated convenience foods. At the end of this chapter you will find a one-week diet plan ideally suited to overweight insomniacs, so if you're going to slim, do it this way.

Overeating is probably even more common a cause of poor sleep than undereating. We have all done it, a special dinner, a night out with friends, a wedding, birthday party, or a meal so good that we didn't want to miss a mouthful – and so to bed – but not to sleep, or at any rate not for long. This time the rumblings are for a different reason. You have to give your poor, abused stomach a chance to deal with that four-course meal you've just stuffed into it, and that takes time. Eating late and going straight to bed would probably not stop you from falling asleep, as for many people eating is a fairly good trigger of the sleep reflexes. Just look around the house after Sunday lunch or Christmas dinner. But as soon as you fall asleep your body's metabolism slows down. This in turn slows down the digestive process, and slow digestion means indigestion. Indigestion leads to discomfort, heartburn and disturbed sleep. Then you're left with the choice of really waking up to find some relief for your complaining innards and probably making a trip to the loo as well, or staying where you are and willing yourself back into a fitful state of somnolence. Either way you're going to lose.

The occasional gastronomic blow-out, followed by a disturbed night, is something we can all live with, but the person who habitually eats late and goes to bed with an overfull stomach may not make the link between their eating habits and the almost inevitable insomnia that will follow. Instead the insomnia itself becomes the focus of their anxieties and they may spend months or years searching for relief from the effect of their bad habits, which they will never find until they remedy the cause.

Social pressures sometimes make it difficult to stand up to your peers and appear to be the odd one out. Business meetings over a meal, large expense accounts, too much alcohol can all become part of ritual behaviour which takes an appalling toll on general health and has a specific effect on sleep. In today's more health-conscious environment more and more restaurants are offering lighter meals and even encouraging customers to eat two or three small starters rather than heavy main courses. Wine waiters no longer sneer when you ask for mineral water; if they do, take your custom somewhere else.

If you're going to eat late at night, copy our Mediterranean neighbours and go for a stroll to help your digestion do its job before you go to bed. If the demands of your job, overtime, shift-work, unsocial hours, are the reason for you getting home late, then remember that this is your leisure time: provided that your work pattern is regularly late nights and late mornings, you can make sure that you have some time to relax after eating and before going to bed. Not only is this socially important, but it will help to override the mental activity that you bring home from the office or factory and replace it with less agitating and disturbing thought-processes.

Fluid consumption is yet another key factor. It's not just what you drink, but how much, that matters. For the proper functioning of the kidneys and urinary system you should consume a minimum of 2½–3 pts (1.5–1.75 litres) of fluid daily, and most of that should be water. Insufficient through-put of liquids can be a cause of recurrent urinary infections and these are an extremely common cause of disturbed sleep, particularly for women. Regular cystitis is a real curse which causes untold misery to millions of women. The continual irritation and burning that it causes, together with the frequency of urination, is a painful and embarrassing problem during the day and a nightmare when you go to bed. Sadly, even when free of the cystitis, the habit of disturbed nights has usually become so ingrained that the beleaguered sufferer still does not enjoy a sound night's sleep.

Coffee, tea and all the sweet fizzy drinks are not suitable substitutes for Adam's ale. They contain caffeine, tannins, sugar and frequently artificial colourings, flavourings and preservatives, all of which can irritate an already sensitive urinary system. These can either aggravate an existing condition of cystitis or can trigger off yet another attack. If you find it difficult to drink large quantities of water, then use diluted pure fruit juices, one quarter juice/three quarters water, or any of the huge selection of herbal teas which are now so easily available. Even the motorway cafés offer a selection, so there's no excuse.

Caffeine is at the root of all sleeping problems for many people, and yet they seem blissfully unaware of the role that this substance plays in keeping them awake. Few parents would encourage their five-, six- or seven-year-olds to drink cups of black coffee, yet I am constantly amazed at how often I see mothers and fathers plying their young children with cola drinks. These all contain caffeine, and caffeine is a substance which irritates the brain. It also occurs in tea and chocolate, and don't forget some of the less obvious sources like coffee or chocolate ice creams, biscuits and cakes.

Caffeinism, or addiction to caffeine, is certainly the commonest form of drug addiction in the western world. If coffee were invented today it's highly unlikely that it would be allowed to be sold to the general public without prescription. Apart from its effects on the central nervous system, it has been linked with raised blood pressure, migraine, breast disease in women, liver problems, stomach ulcers and other digestive problems. Too much of it causes tremors in the hands and fingers, and depriving the addict of a regular 'fix' can cause uncomfortable withdrawal symptoms, particularly severe headaches and the shakes.

The human race being what it is, we all know people who drink three large espresso coffees after dinner and instantly fall asleep in the armchair. But for most people caffeine is an important cause of insomnia. Incidentally, it is also a powerful diuretic, so that even if you are not kept awake by your increased brain activity, the regular trips to the bathroom make sure that you don't sleep too well if you drink coffee late at night. Some people are extremely sensitive to caffeine and for them more than a cup or two in the morning can affect their sleep at night.

There are plenty of substitutes and extremely good decaffeinated coffees and teas. Some people seem to be worried about the chemicals used during the decaffeinating process, but nearly all of the well known brand names use steam to remove the caffeine from the beans, so there is no need to worry.

Many prescribed and over-the-counter medicines contain stimulants, so if you are having problems with your sleep do check with your doctor and pharmacist in case any of the drugs which you are taking could be the cause of your problem. Thyroid drugs, oral contraceptives, beta-blockers and many headache and cold-cure remedies fall into this category, as do some of the illegal drugs like marijuana and cocaine.

Alcohol can play an important role which is often misunderstood. Very small quantities such as half a pub measure of spirits or half a glass of wine may have a mildly sedative effect, but larger quantities of alcohol can seriously interfere with sleep. People who consistently drink large quantities of alcohol tend to have predominantly shallow sleep and alcoholics also suffer a disruption of their dreaming patterns. They tend to have their dreams during the daytime in the form of hallucinations. Too much alcohol also interferes with eating habits and destroys some of the B vitamins which are vital substances for proper sleep as well as for ensuring the general health and functioning of the human body.

The idea of 'sleeping it off' is also a misnomer. Far from helping, the prolonged stuporous sleep of the hangover is not natural sleep and does not conform to the normal patterns. What's more the consequences can be serious or even fatal. Under the influence of alcohol you are less likely to move during your sleep, so that it is possible to do serious and sometimes irreversible damage to nerves which get compressed by the weight of the body. Inhaled vomit is a frequent cause of death related to alcohol abuse. The drunk does not even wake up when he throws up.

The combination of alcohol and sleeping pills is probably the most common abuse resorted to by the insomniac and, whilst alcohol does enhance the effect of sleeping pills, all that happens is that you get off to sleep more easily but you are just putting off the problems till later in the night, when you are likely to wake up and not get back to sleep again.

Exercise can help or hinder your sleep. An evening game of squash might be good aerobic exercise and help to keep you fit, but the very nature of the game is aggressive and, in common with other competitive sports, can produce enormous outpourings of adrenalin which is a powerful stimulant. Some sports can create considerable emotional stress. How many golfers amongst you lie in bed and replay every shot after a bad round, or worse still rehash the one missed putt which cost you the game, over and over again? Exercise should be beneficial and leave you feeling both physically and mentally relaxed and comfortable, but it all depends on your attitude to the game you are playing.

Don't play to win, but rather, play for the pure enjoyment of the game and of using your body. If you can change your attitude so that you are less competitive, but still put your all into the sport, your enjoyment will be on a very different level, your body will produce less adrenalin, and sleep will come much easier. It doesn't matter whether you enjoy walking, swimming, cycling, bowls or hang-gliding, the magic word is enjoy. If you exercise as a ritual penance and your attitude is that of doing something you have to do or ought to do, rather than something you really want to do, then you will be frustrated when you don't succeed, resentful of the time you spend and agitated when you go to bed.

Bedtime habits should all steer you towards slipping between the sheets, or under the duvet, in a calm, peaceful and relaxed frame of mind. To this end don't fall into the trap of making bedtime the period of the day when you and your partner discuss contentious issues or argue over the housekeeping or the kids' behaviour. This may sound like stating the obvious, but for many couples this may be the only time in the 24 hours when there are no other demands and distractions. This is a definite no-no, as it guarantees sleepless nights, probably for both of you, and it's also not likely to be very good for your sex life. Sex can play an important role in encouraging good sleep and anything which gets in the way of the physical side of your loving relationships should be avoided at all costs.

Try to get into the habit of setting aside time earlier in the evening to talk to each other. It's not as hard as it sounds, it just needs a little planning and discipline. Going to bed on unresolved problems and frustrations will keep your mind turning till the small hours, so sort out your differences by talking to each other. So often partners expect their other halves to be psychic and to understand and anticipate their problems and difficulties, but sadly few of us have the good fortune to have a medium in the family.

Don't forget your children in this respect. Adults seldom recognise that children, too, have problems and anxieties that need resolving, and they are no less likely to suffer from insomnia than you are. In this age of technology with TVs, videos, computers and all the other electronic wizardry that fills our homes, we all need to be careful not to let the machines take over. If your child seems anxious or upset, discuss things and make sure that you do it when you both have time. It's no good starting on a difficult conversation when one or other of you is dashing for the school bus or the morning train to the office. Don't dismiss a child's worries about not being liked by teachers, not keeping up with the class or having difficulties making friends. These fears are very real and very disturbing to a young child or teenager, and are frequently the root of sleeping disorders which can become habitual and pose a problem for the rest of their lives.

Any major event in life can upset your nocturnal habits. Bereavement, redundancy, moving home, getting married, being pregnant, having a baby, taking exams, going for interviews, even travelling and jet lag can all take their toll. If your bedtime routine is always the same, the rituals become comforting and help to push the anxieties out of focus. Get into the habit of doing things in a fixed routine. For instance, get undressed, wash, put on your pyjamas, clean your teeth, check that all the lights are out, pull the plug out of the television set, do two or three minutes of relaxation exercises, get into bed, read for five minutes, turn the light out and go to sleep. You'll find a routine that suits you, and once you do, stick to it, even when you travel. Be careful about the book you read: a romantic novel or a book of poems is more likely to lull you off than the latest Wilbur Smith adventure story, which will keep you on the edge of the bed.

For most people sitting up late and watching horror movies, westerns or thrillers is also not ideal. If you really want a technological sleeping pill why not keep a tape of *The Sound of Music* in the video machine?

One problem with rituals is that sometimes you are forced to change them. If you've always gone to bed with your favourite teddy, you might worry that your new wife would find it odd, so you leave it at home with Mum, but then you can't sleep! If you've always slept in nothing but Chanel No. 5, you might think a sexy nightie more appropriate for a new wife, which is fine till it ruckles up round your neck and you think it's strangling you in the night.

Probably the most important single factor is the bed you sleep in. As an osteopath I am constantly amazed by how many people buy a bed when they get married and are still sleeping in the same one 20 years later. In that period the average family has changed their car seven times, the television three times, the fridge twice, the washing machine twice, the sitting-room furniture at least once, the lawnmower often, and yet they stick to the same sagging, lumpy bed.

Even if you don't get backache as a result of this monstrosity, you are certainly going to roll into the crater in the middle, or on to the side of the heavier partner. Never one to discourage close companionship in bed, I still maintain that it is much better both for your back and for your sexual relationships to be on a firm, level and supported mattress. Backache is a serious cause of sleep loss, and bad beds are a serious cause of backache. If you can't afford to change your bed, then at least put a sheet of plywood under the mattress. This should be not less than 4 in (10 cm) narrower than the bed and 1 ft (30 cm) shorter. Do make sure you wrap the board in an old sheet or thin blanket, otherwise the corners will make holes in the bottom of your mattress, and watch out for your finger nails when you're tucking the sheet under the mattress.

Pillows are another important factor. Get into the habit of sleeping as flat as possible – one small pillow is all you need, and unless you are allergic to feathers buy the best feather pillow you can afford. You can mould a good pillow to fit into the shape of your head and neck and support you where you need it. Synthetic foam pillows are too firm, and your head bounces around on the top like the plastic duck in your bath.

Acquire the habit of sleeping in a cool room with some ventilation. Hot stuffy bedrooms block up your nose and sinuses, dry out your mucous membranes and wake you in the middle of the night with a sore throat, a headache or a tickly cough. In winter time make sure that you have humidifiers on your radiators, or at least hang a wet towl over them before you go to bed. This is particularly important for asthmatics or bronchitics as warm moist air is less likely to irritate the airways of the lungs and trigger off bouts of coughing or attacks of asthma.

For the chronic insomniac one of the best habits to acquire is any one of the relaxation techniques – yoga, meditation, biofeedback, relaxation exercises or self-hypnosis (see Chapter 9).

If you need to lose weight or if you just want to lose a few pounds to get into your summer swimsuit, then as we've seen already, how you do it is very important in relation to your sleep problem. Here is a one-week diet plan which I have used with great success for my patients for many years.

Apart from the first day, you won't be hungry. In fact most people find that they can't eat all the food that is on the diet. You can switch whole days around within the week except for the first day, and you can switch meals around within each day.

This eating plan is not designed as a weight-loss regime but as a spring clean and tonic for the whole system. Try to start on a day when you can take things fairly gently; after that you'll have no problem following your normal lifestyle. At the end of seven days you will feel really great and the bonus is that if you needed to lose weight, you will have done so.

You can consume as much water or weak tea without sugar as you like, but in any case your total fluid intake should be 2½–3 pts (1.5–1.75 litres) each day.

You should take two 5 ml teaspoons of Bio-Strath Elixir before each meal. This is a general tonic which helps your metabolism to function well, encourages the absorption of nutrients from your food and helps to increase your natural resistance to disease and infection.

Don't worry about the calories, there are certainly far more than you would normally expect on a weight loss diet. Follow this plan as closely as you can, but if for any reason you fall by the wayside one day, don't give up! All you need to do is to repeat the day on which you overindulged, but this time stick to the diet.

You can make a healthy and delicious dressing for all the salads in this week with three parts extra virgin olive oil to one part cider vinegar. Add a pinch of dried mustard, a finely chopped clove of garlic, two finely chopped spring onions, a sprinkle of herbes de provence, and black pepper.

1st Day

Breakfast

2 (5ml) teaspoons of Bio-Strath
1 glass of fruit or vegetable juice
1 portion of natural yoghurt

Lunch

2 (5ml) teaspoons of Bio-Strath
1 glass of fruit juice and 1 glass of vegetable juice
1 portion of yoghurt

Supper

2 (5ml) teaspoons of Bio-Strath
1 glass of fruit or vegetable juice
1 portion of yoghurt
1 cup of herb tea (e.g. Solidago) or weak Indian tea without sugar

2nd Day

Breakfast

Standard Breakfast consisting of:
2 (5ml) teaspoons of Bio-Strath
1 fruit
1 to 2 slices of wholemeal bread with cottage cheese
1 portion of natural yoghurt
1 cup of weak tea or skimmed milk

Lunch

2 (5ml) teaspoons of Bio-Strath
1 fruit
about 7 oz (200 gm) of raw vegetable salad
about 10 oz (280 gm) of steamed vegetables with one spoon of sunflower oil

Supper

2 (5 ml) teaspoons of Bio-Strath
1 fruit
5 oz (140 gm) of muesli mixed with yoghurt
1 cup of weak tea

3rd Day

Breakfast

Standard Breakfast (as on 2nd day)

Lunch

2 (5 ml) teaspoons of Bio-Strath
1 fruit
7 oz (200 gm) of mixed salad

1 jacket potato with about 2 oz (55 gm) of cottage cheese with herbs

Supper

2 (5ml) teaspoons of Bio-Strath
1 portion of yoghurt with fruit added
1 slice of wholemeal bread with low fat cheese
1 cup of weak tea

4th Day – Rice Day

The total quantity of rice for the day should be prepared in the morning (3 oz/90 gm of dry rice cooked in ¼ pt (0.5 litre) water or vegetable broth will produce 7–8oz/ 200–230 gm).

Breakfast

2 (5 ml) teaspoons of Bio-Strath
5 oz (140 gm) of boiled rice
5 oz (140 gm) of stewed apple sweetened with honey and flavoured with cinnamon and grated lemon rind

Lunch

2 (5 ml) teaspoons of Bio-Strath
About 7 oz (200 gm) of boiled rice
7 oz (200 gm) of steamed vegetables (tomatoes, celery, etc.)

Supper

2 (5ml) teaspoons of Bio-Strath
5 oz (140 gm) of boiled rice
5 oz (140 gm) of orange (fleshy part only)

5th Day

Breakfast

Standard Breakfast (as on 2nd and 3rd days)

Lunch

2 (5 ml) teaspoons of Bio-Strath
1 fruit
about 7 oz (200 gm) of raw vegetable salad
1 jacket potato
about 3 oz (90 gm) of steamed spinach without sauce but mixed with 1 (25 ml) tablespoon of sunflower oil

Supper

2 (5 ml) teaspoons of Bio-Strath
5 oz (140 gm) of cottage cheese mixed to a cream with sour milk and poured over chopped fruit
1 cup of weak tea

6th Day

Breakfast

Standard Breakfast (as on 2nd, 3rd and 5th days)

Lunch

2 (5 ml) teaspoons of Bio-Strath
1 fruit
7 oz (200 gm) of mixed salad
1 jacket potato
about 3 oz (90 gm) of steamed beans with 1 (25 ml) tablespoonful of sunflower oil

Supper

2 (5 ml) teaspoons of Bio-Strath
1 fruit
5 oz (140 gm) of muesli mixed with yoghurt
1 or 2 slices of wholemeal bread with low fat cheese
1 cup of weak tea

7th Day

Breakfast

Standard Breakfast (as on 2nd, 3rd, 5th and 6th days)

Lunch

2 (5 ml) teaspoons of Bio-Strath
1 fruit
7 oz (200 gm) of mixed salad
a choice of: blue trout (steamed in aluminium foil and served with chopped parsley and lemon juice) or grilled chopped veal cutlets or vegetarian soya cutlet with boiled potatoes
1 fruit salad

Supper

2 (5 ml) teaspoons of Bio-Strath
1 fruit and a choice of a lightly boiled egg and

1 or 2 slices of wholemeal bread, or ham, cheese and wholemeal bread (with a little butter)
1 cup of weak tea

Well done! You have finished your diet week. You have probably lost a few pounds and certainly feel great. You can safely repeat this diet several times a year and in any case it's a good idea for the family to pick one day out of the diet and stick to it once a week.

3

SLEEP: ORDER AND DISORDER

'Insomnia never comes to a man who has to get up exactly at six o'clock. Insomnia troubles only those who can sleep any time.'

Elbert G. Hubbard

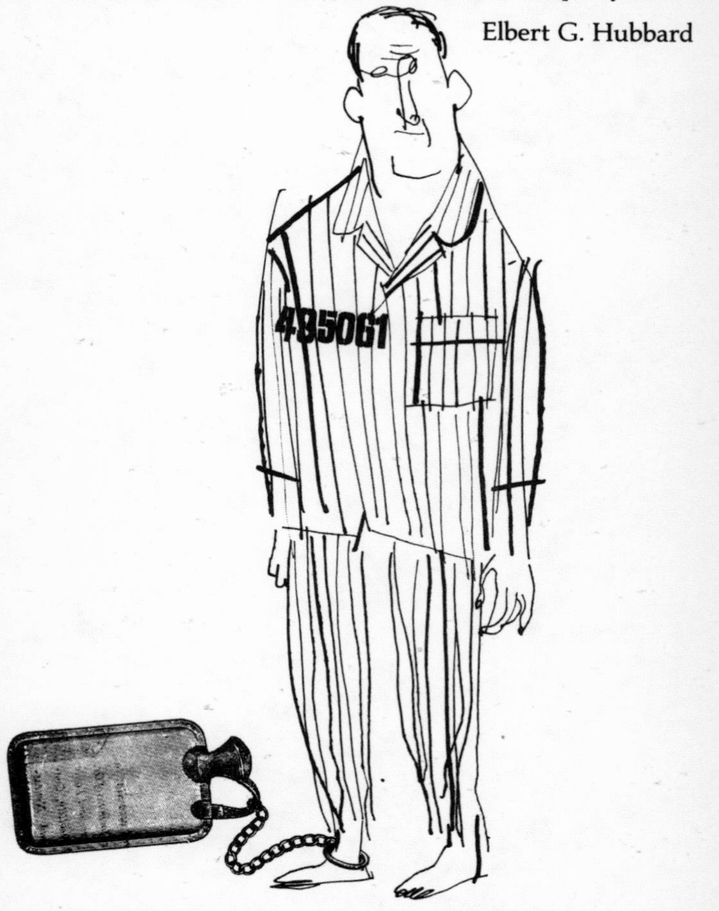

This quotation may seem rather trite, especially to those cursed with insomnia. There is considerably more than a grain of truth in it, though. The American humorist James Thurber was quoted as saying, 'Early to rise and early to bed makes a male healthy, wealthy and dead', but nothing could be further from the truth: in fact, the original proverb points us in the right direction for better sleep.

It may sound boring and unadventurous, but developing regular habits of going to bed and getting up is of paramount importance if you're going to deal with your problem. As with so many of the tips and ideas throughout this book, do not expect perfect sleep after trying this for just two or three days. Re-educating your sleep patterns is a slow business and you will see only slow results. It is essential that you persevere if you want to achieve long-term benefits. But you have to *want* to. Before you embark on making changes to your lifestyle and putting theory into practice, perhaps this is an opportune moment to reflect on your own motives. Do you really want to be a better sleeper? Do you in fact suffer from insomnia? Is your insomnia real, imagined (just as real), or invented (not real at all) – a cry for help or a ploy for getting more attention? Is it a handy excuse for underachievement or a means of avoiding blame or responsibility? Do you need your insomnia as a way of preserving your image of a haggard, drawn, dedicated and overworked parent, doctor, social worker, business executive or foreman? Do you find it easier than the proverbial headache as a means of avoiding sex? In other words, do you want to get better or would you rather be a lifelong insomniac?

These may seem like harsh words, and if I've offended you I hope you will forgive me. I pose these questions so that you can answer them in order to help identify and solve the problem. If you are an insomniac it doesn't matter what the cause is, so long as you can identify it, and the same applies if you are a pseudo-insomniac. The only thing I ask of you is that you are honest with yourself. You can fool everyone else, and contrary to popular belief it is possible to fool all of the people all of the time. If you answer these questions honestly you will soon find out whether you are also fooling yourself. If you are, now's the time to do something about it.

As we've seen in Chapter 1, one of the main physiological differences that occurs during our circadian cycle is the rise and fall of body temperature, and this has a vital role to play in whether we feel sleepy or awake. Studies on students who traditionally lead fairly erratic lives, going to parties, sitting up talking into the small hours, cramming for exams and staying in bed till midday when they have no lectures to attend, have shown that these irregular livers have a much smaller difference between their lowest and highest body temperatures and a less regular pattern to the times of day and night when they felt more alert or more sleepy.

Comparisons between the irregular students and a group who led more ordered lives produced surprising differences. Those who consistently went to bed and got up at roughly the same time tended to feel more satisfied with life and more energetic; they performed better in physical tests designed to measure concentration and reaction times. These studies confirm what the families of shift-workers and the workers themselves have known for years, namely that their sleep is not so refreshing and that they tend to feel constantly lacking in energy.

Whatever the reasons for your insomnia one effect is common to all sufferers. Insomnia disturbs your biological time clock. This clock is a reflex pattern to which the body becomes conditioned; a disrupted sleep routine imposes changes on the clock which eventually becomes conditioned to fit in with your disturbed sleep patterns. In effect the tail is wagging the dog – or perhaps it should be the sheep in the case of insomnia. Like all conditioned reflexes they can be changed by training, and reprogramming your biological time clock is the prime requirement of any attempt to manage your life better so that you can restore your body to normal sleeping and waking functions.

The first thing you must do is to go out and buy the largest, loudest, nastiest alarm clock you can find. It is pointless getting a genteel bleep, a snooze facility or worst of all a clock that stops buzzing when you shout at it. You need a good old-fashioned tin clock with two bells and a hammer which makes enough noise to wake the dead. The next thing you need is an old biscuit tin large enough for the clock to stand in. The reasons will become apparent in a moment.

Now plan your life for the next three or four weeks. Refuse all social engagements which are going to keep you out too late. Avoid situations of over-excitement, over-anxiety or excessive tension, especially those that occur during the evening. Acquire a selection of good light reading – Barbara Cartland or Mills and Boon are ideal bedtime books. They're undemanding, romantic and hardly over stimulating.

Tell your family and all your friends what you are planning to do. This will avoid one o'clock in the morning phone calls from someone wanting a chat, and unwelcome visits from those popping in for a late night cup of coffee and a brandy; this type of visit never seems to end before two in the morning.

Decide on a time that you are going to go to bed – for argument's sake let's say 10 p.m. Regardless of how tired or otherwise you feel, go to bed at exactly that time every night. Follow a routine, turn off the TV, make yourself a cup of Horlicks, take it to the bedroom, get undressed, run the bath and have a good ten-minute soak using one of the relaxing herbal oils (see page 94), clean your teeth, put on your pyjamas or not as the case may be, go to bed, read, listen to gentle music – not the late night news – turn the light out and go to sleep.

But what about the alarm clock? Before you finally get into bed put the clock into the biscuit tin on a table just out of reach. Even if you have no need to get up in the morning, set the clock for the same time every single day, preferably early, and when it rings get up, don't doze, don't dally, don't take an extra five minutes – just get up instantly.

Why should you get up at six o'clock in the morning when you're not going to work that day, or you're on holiday, or you're out of work? You are going to get up at six o'clock because the sooner you establish a routine of early waking, the sooner your body clock will start to tell you that you feel tired at a sensible time in the evening. When you go to bed feeling tired, you'll go to sleep quickly.

Follow this routine for at least a month. Don't break it, don't vary it, don't sit up to watch something 'special' on the telly. Bit by bit these regular habits will override the disrupted biological clock which you have acquired through your bad habits, and by the end of the month your body should be well established in the new routine of your biological clock ticking away as it should be, in harmony with day and night.

Some people will respond to this rigorous discipline very quickly, and others may take longer, but just because you find that your sleeping improves in the first week or two don't be lulled into a sense of false security. The old habits will come back very quickly if you let them. The longer you persevere with this seemingly draconian regime, the more firmly established the conditioned reflex patterns of your new time clock become. As time goes by you will naturally want to have the odd late night out or in front of the telly, but do be sure to introduce changes very gradually to begin with. No matter what time you go to bed, get up at your regular time next morning. If you've had a serious problem with your sleep it is likely to come back more easily if you start abusing your time clock. It's worth being as rigid as you can about your getting up time and, providing you don't have a week of late nights on the trot, you will have no ill effects other than feeling a bit more tired the next day, following the occasional night out.

Depression is frequently cited as being both cause and effect of sleep disorders. There is no doubt that poor quality sleep is often an early symptom of the onset of depression, and as anyone who suffers from chronically bad sleep will know, endless nights of tossing and turning or sitting up in front of the television are bound to have a depressive effect. If you seem to fit into either of these categories, cheer up because there is some good news.

Recent research by Professor Jim Horne in California makes a link between too much sleep and depression. In his sleep laboratory Horne has studied the effects of reducing the amount of sleep in patients suffering from severe depression. By waking them after four or five hours, he found that many of the depressive patients felt much better the next day. Not surprisingly, they felt rather tired – but not depressed. The same patients left to sleep for eight hours felt a return of their depression as soon as they got up.

What frequently happens to depressive insomniacs is that their biological time-clock is disrupted and though they may not sleep during the night, it's likely that they will have too much sleep during the daylight hours. Helping to relieve depression could be one additional benefit of learning to regulate your sleeping time. This is one more reason for making sure that whatever time you go to bed you keep your alarm clock set to the same hour every morning.

Getting order back into your sleeping habits is one thing; trying to eliminate some of the disorder can be rather more difficult. Some disorder might be unavoidable – jet lag, shift-work, caring for the sick or occasional late-night social commitments. Avoidable disorder is within your own control – smoking, alcohol, lack of exercise, pointless anger and your own personal sleeping conditions.

No-one who smokes can possibly be unaware of the serious health hazards which indulging in this habit entails. What few smokers, or for that matter their doctors, know is that smoking can seriously damage your sleep. The main effects of nicotine are to increase the heart rate and blood pressure, and to raise the body's state of arousal (it's the heightened arousal effect for which most people continue to smoke).

Studies at Pennsylvania State University compared the length of time which it took smokers and non-smokers to get to sleep. In general, the smokers took twice as long. In volunteers who agreed to stop smoking, the time which it took them to get to sleep fell from an average of 52 minutes whilst they were smoking to only 18 minutes within two nights of quitting the weed. If you must smoke, don't have your last cigarette just before bedtime – or, worse still, after you've slid between the sheets. If you're determined to solve your sleep problem and can't give up the cigarettes, then at least try not to smoke for one hour before bedtime.

Another good reason for giving up smoking is that nicotine is a vaso-constrictor; that is, it reduces the diameter of blood vessels, one side effect of which is to reduce the size of the male erection. Since sexual satisfaction is one of the great relievers of insomnia, giving up now could double the chances of better sleep for you and your partner. Caffeine has the same effect. According to Voltaire, coffee is the drink of eunuchs – who obviously had no such considerations on their minds.

Of all the popular misconceptions that abound in the area of sleep disorders, the idea that alcohol helps to overcome these problems – or indeed that it is better to have a hot toddy (or two, or three) or half a bottle of wine, or three pints of your favourite brew than it is to take a sleeping pill – is perhaps the furthest from the truth.

Taking moderate amounts of alcohol may help you to get to sleep quicker, but it's quite likely to disturb the pattern of your sleep and to shorten periods of paradoxical sleep during the first part of the night. If you have considerably more alcohol than you are used to, then there is an increased risk of what is called a rebound effect. This happens because alcohol is broken down rapidly in the body and by the small hours it will have been eliminated, leaving you awake, thirsty and hung-over, a feeling likely to last well into the next day. An added danger is that you feel so awful that you're tempted to take a hair of the dog. The alcohol abuser wakes from sleep trembling, anxious and desperate for the next drink. The dividing line between the insomniac drinking larger quantities and more frequently in a vain attempt to improve their sleeping, and the confirmed alcoholic, is very fine and extremely easy to cross. If you want a bedtime nightcap stick to the sedative herbal teas (see page 89) or one of the popular malted milk drinks (see page 109).

The idea that exercise improves sleep is another of the old wives' tales which most mothers pass on to their children. This one is basically true, though it does depend on a number of factors. In the affluent world of the late 20th century few of us get sufficient exercise without making a specific effort to do so. More and more jobs are sedentary; even the traditionally manual occupations are becoming more mechanised; and an ever-increasing part of our leisure time is spent sitting in cars or rooted to the armchair in front of the television.

This type of lifestyle does not encourage sound, refreshing and regenerating sleep. The answer is to incorporate regular physical activity into your everyday life. Trained athletes show an increase in both the quality and quantity of their sleep. What does not help are sudden bursts of infrequent but intensive physical activity. This sort of exercise will only serve to increase the heart rate, body temperature and adrenalin production so that you go to bed in an over-heated, over-excited state of both mind and body. Pick an activity which you enjoy, start gently and build up to a regular and reasonably strenuous regime – but don't let it become an obsession. Regular exercise increases the amount of growth hormone produced during the night (see page 12), and this encourages deeper sleep in Stage 4 (see page 14).

Another good reason for regular exercise is that it is an excellent way of dissipating the anger and frustrations of the day. It uses up the excess amounts of adrenalin which your body has manufactured in response to the fright, fight and flight reflex (see page 13). Going to bed in a state of unresolved anger or bitterness does not help your sleep, and rehashing every pinprick or the slings and arrows that life has hurled at you during the day helps even less.

As the night progresses and repose eludes you it's inevitable that your anger will intensify, your feelings of injury will be magnified and your mental plottings to get even, to get your own back, to make 'them' pay for it will churn around in your mind, banishing sleep forever – or at least for what feels like forever. Getting off this merry-go-round is your first priority. You need a conscious effort to put these destructive thoughts and emotions out of your mind. Try some of the relaxation techniques (see page 122). These will help you to get to sleep before the nagging hurt in the back of your mind becomes an unstoppable tide of negative feelings.

Creating order in the bedroom is one of the key factors in overcoming your problems. This does not mean developing an obsession for neatness and tidiness, but evolving a practical system which will suit your individual needs for comfort, which is the prerequisite for sleep. Sometimes, if insomnia is a comparatively recent experience, it is worth trying to think back to a period in life when your sleep was good. Try to identify what was different at that time. Did you have a bed that was harder or softer? Larger or smaller? Were you facing the door? Were you sleeping north-south rather than east-west? Did you use a duvet or did you sleep in a bed with three heavy blankets and tightly tucked hospital corners? Maybe, during your good sleeping period, your bedroom was warmer or cooler than the one you have now.

All these variables may play an important part in overcoming your present difficulties. Most people sleep better in firm rather than soft beds, most in cooler rather than warmer bedrooms and most with lighter rather than heavier bedding (especially if there is central heating). But remember that these 'mosts' may not apply to you. What suits you is what suits you, and once you've found what it is, stick to it.

This can sometimes lead to insurmountable problems within a relationship. If one partner needs the windows open, no pyjamas and a thin cotton sheet to enjoy sleep on a rock hard bed, and the other wants to wallow in a soft mattress, swathed in wincyette and enveloped in the highest-rated duvet and an electric blanket you are in trouble. It's probably better to solve the sleeping problems first and then try to sort out the relationship.

Technically speaking, firmer beds give better support, better sleep and less risk of back problems. Room temperatures of less than 70°F (21°C) – –60°F (15°C) if you are asthmatic, as the house-dust mite can't survive below this temperature and the droppings of this creature are one of the most powerful allergens – are generally the most acceptable. Curtains or blinds which exclude daylight can help to prevent early morning wakening, especially in the summer.

Disorder caused by jet lag, shift-work or other anti-social working patterns is one of the hardest of all problems to overcome (see page 13). Some of the latest experiments conducted by Dr Charles Czeisler at Harvard Medical School have reinforced earlier work by pioneers in the field of light therapy.

The hormone melatonin is a body chemical which helps to induce sleep. It has been known for many years that this hormone is produced according to the presence or absence of daylight, and is a key factor in inducing the state of hibernation in animals. As daylight hours get less and the hours of darkness increase, more melatonin is produced, the body's physiological functions slow down, animals put on weight and finally go to sleep for the rest of the winter.

It has already been established that the 'winter blues' or SAD – seasonal affective disorder – can be successfully treated by exposure to high intensity light. Dr Czeisler exposed volunteers to brightly lit screens while they worked through the night, then sent them to bed in totally blacked-out rooms. Within four nights they had adjusted to the reversal of day and night, unlike a second group who had worked all night in conventional lighting and whose bedrooms were fitted with normal curtains.

The bright-light volunteers reversed the normal patterns of body temperature and hormone production (see page 12), whereas the others were still functioning on the natural circadian rhythm with all the problems that entails for night-workers.

Jet lag can be overcome in the same way – by influencing the body's production of melatonin. Exposure to high-intensity light or getting extra bright daylight exposure when you arrive at your destination will both help. The use of melatonin in drug form is also being tried experimentally, and early work at the University of Surrey has shown promising results.

Looking out of your kitchen window on to a sunlit garden you are seeing a light intensity of 2000 lux. A Mediterranean beach at midday is 5000 lux and the average office or factory environment is around 500 lux. Improving the levels of illumination in the workplace and at home, particularly during the winter months, can have a highly beneficial effect, both on preventing depression and improving sleep.

If you can find the order which encourages you to enjoy good, sound, refreshing, restoring and regular sleep, you will have found the key to making an all-round improvement a reality. If you can resolve the disorder which has chronically interfered with your ability to go to sleep when you want to and wake up when you need to, feeling eager to face the day, you will have cleared the first and most difficult hurdle in the race to somnolence.

4

TO SLEEP, PERCHANCE TO DREAM – NIGHTMARES AND NIGHT TERRORS

'With thousand such enchanting dreams, that meet to make sleep not so sound, as sweet.'

Robert Herrick

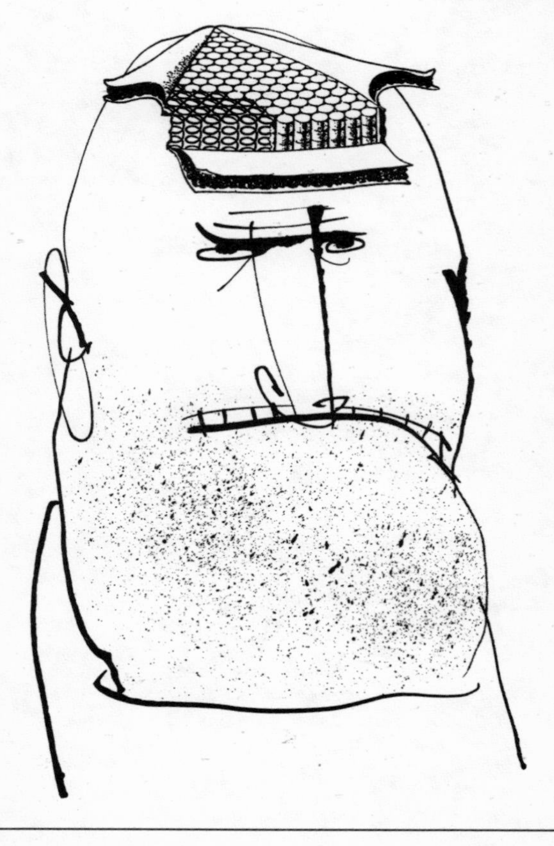

Long before modern scientists, psychiatrists and psychologists started to explore the significance of dreams, philosophers, poets, musicians and soothsayers not only understood the beauty and importance of our dreams, but some of them learned to manipulate the interpretation of dreams, often with remarkable outcomes.

In this chapter we shall explore together the mystical pathways into the world of sleep and dreams. We shall try to explain and find remedies for bad dreams, nightmares and night terrors. We shall investigate the strange phenomena of sleep-talking and sleep-walking. We shall assess the impact of all these factors on both quality and quantity of sleep, and explore ways to utilise dreams, to encourage good dreams and compensate for the negative aspects of our less desirable sleep occurrences.

In spite of the scientists' explanations of how and why we dream, the 'prophetic dream theory' still has a huge following. Quite apart from the psychoanalytical approach, first developed by Freud, there is still a thriving industry which revolves around dream interpretation. Whether true or false, quackery, opportunism or just plain coincidence, dreams and their interpretation have undoubtedly shaped the destiny of nations as well as people.

When the Pharaoh dreamed of 'seven fat and seven lean kine' and 'seven full and seven empty ears of corn', Joseph claimed that these dreams foretold seven years of plenty and seven years of famine. How right he was, and his explanation of the Pharaoh's dreams saved his life and the nation. Imagine the next 2000 years of history without Joseph and the other 11 sons of Jacob. Without the dreams of Achilles before the battle of Troy, of Julius Caesar, Joan of Arc, Napoleon, Alexander the Great and Hitler, how different a place the world would be.

Nerys Dee, in *The Dreamer's Workbook*, describes how one

nightmare changed the course of modern history with world-shattering consequences. In November 1917, with the German and French armies on opposite sides of the Somme, Adolf Hitler, then a corporal, woke from a terrifying nightmare in which he was crushed by debris. He dashed out into the night; seconds later a shell fell on his bunker and killed everyone in it. If it hadn't been for that nightmare . . .?

Many primitive peoples have made use of dreams and dream interpretation as part of their cultural heritage. The North American Indians and the Aborigines both valued and treasured their dreams. It was common practice in ancient Greece, India, Japan and Egypt, deliberately to encourage dreams. To this end special shrines were built where dreams could be 'incubated'. Petitioners lay on stone beds within the shrine, and the messengers of the gods would bring help and healing through sleep and dreams. The oracle at Delphi and the temple at Epidauros can still be visited today. Nobody who has stood in either can fail to feel 'something' in the air.

The poems of Homer, the earliest surviving Greek texts, refer to dreams as a form of revelation. Plato tells us that while awaiting execution Socrates was writing poems as instructed in his dreams. Plato foreshadowed Freud by centuries when he described the frequently reported dreams of incest as being nothing more than wish fulfilment, when most of his contemporaries thought of them as being important symbols of things to come. At one time, early in his writings, Aristotle explained dreams as the result of soul using clairvoyant powers once it was freed from its earthly body whilst its owner slept.

In today's scientific and technological world, it is perhaps more difficult to believe in Hypnos the god of sleep, Morpheus the god of dreams and Hermes the messenger as the source of our dreams. Maybe those ancient beliefs enabled our forefathers to open their minds, allowing the seemingly limitless power of the human brain to compute all the variables in a given situation and come up with a print-out of the best possible solution. Is it feasible that we all have within us solutions to our problems and difficulties, but lack the will, commitment or ability to face the execution of those solutions consciously? By preparing for sleep and encouraging good dreaming, can we learn to free our subconscious from its constraints and liberate its creative ability to the full?

If so, we must also learn to capture the memory of our dreams.

The step from sorcery to science came with Sigmund Freud in his book *The Interpretation of Dreams*, published in 1900. After working for some years with hypnosis, a therapy with which he became increasingly disenchanted, Freud developed a technique known as free association, which he used in his work on the interpretation of his patients' dreams. He encouraged them to relax and let their minds drift, undirected, from dream sequences to reality, memories or emotions. This, claimed Freud, enabled him to use the remembered story of the dream to lead the patient to the underlying desires which triggered the dream. For he was certain that these were distant recollections and fantasies to the deep emotions of infancy. Dreams, he said, are infantile wish fulfilment expressed during sleep. In later life, and in the light of working on the problem of recurrent dreams, particularly in the field of war neuroses, Freud did modify his theories and accepted that there were some dreams which did not fit his original concept.

The sexual connotations of Freud's work caused a considerable furore in early 20th century circles and have continued to be the subject of heated debate ever since. Nonetheless even the scientists mostly accept that dreaming is a manifestation of man's creativity, although few of them would go along with the dream prophecy theory.

A more interesting explanation of some of our esoteric and bizarre dreams can be found in the writings of Carl Gustav Jung, a Swiss psychologist who for some years worked quite closely with Freud. There was one fundamental difference in their beliefs. Jung developed the concept of the Collective Unconscious and the archetypal images through which it is manifest. He believed that man inherited subconscious images from his predecessors and it was these images, buried deep in the subconscious, which surfaced in dreams. This, he explains, is why many mythological subjects occur in the dreams of those who can have had no knowledge of that particular mythology. He describes many patients who had dreams containing similar stories to myths and legends from distant traditions. He even cites his own experience when going through a severe mid-life crisis. He took up painting as an outlet for his frustrations and on impulse started to produce abstract designs which frequently seemed to end as circles divided into four, or multiples of four. It was years later that he found similar designs known as 'mandala' used throughout the east as an alternative to the spoken 'mantra' (see page 129), as an aid to meditation in yoga.

Jung believed fervently that we all inherited memories from our ancestral past, possibly even on a global scale. If this is so, it is no wonder that our dreams can be so remarkable.

What's in a dream?

Sometimes dreams are so totally different from our everyday conscious experiences that it is tempting to explain them by the presence of aliens or the departure of the soul. In truth they are brief episodes of fantasy when we feel emotions, when we do things, when things happen to us, and when people, animals or mythological creatures join in. We often dream in colour, though people blind from birth see nothing in their dreams although in every other way the dreams are just as vivid as those of the sighted. Dreams are short bursts of madness which inhabit our sleeping hours.

Research has shown that we all dream, even though you may be one of those who never remember yours or think that you are the exception. During the 1950s and '60s, Drs Kleitman and Dement tried waking up volunteers at different periods during their sleep and asking them questions about their dreams. Their findings were surprising. Eighty per cent of those wakened just as their eyes had started rapid movements – that is at the beginning of periods of paradoxical sleep – said they had been dreaming. Only 7% of those woken out of orthodox sleep were dreaming at the time. Dreams do occur during orthodox sleep but, apart from the fantastic dreams which are common in the very first stages of sleep, the majority of exciting dreams happen during paradoxical sleep; most that occur during orthodox sleep tend towards the mundane. In 1962 studies by David Foulkes in Chicago confirmed this. Instead of asking his volunteers 'Have you been dreaming?', he asked, 'What was passing through your mind?' The answers revealed almost as much recall from orthodox as from paradoxical sleep. But his subjects tended to describe the mundane happenings as thinking rather than dreaming.

In all cases what became apparent was how quickly the ability to recall dreams vanishes. Allowing this to happen is a great shame. Remembering your dreams, even the unpleasant ones, can be a powerful insight into situations, anxieties, unresolved problems, sexuality and emotional stresses which could be interfering with your sleep. On an even more positive note, dream sequences are highly creative and can be a boon to playwrights, novelists, scriptwriters, as they provide a rich vein of imaginary scenarios which arise unfettered by conscious constraints and predetermined thought-processes. For all these reasons you should acquire the habit of keeping a detailed dream book.

'How can I, I never remember what I've dreamt?' I hear you cry. Don't worry, you can learn to remember your dreams and once you start to record them you will find it a fascinating, rewarding and helpful process. It's a simple thing to do. It requires only the will to do it, a little practice and the self-discipline to stick to a routine. Make sure that you have a notebook and pencil, and a light which is easy to switch on, beside your bed at all times. Pencils are better than pens as they are more reliable, don't have caps you have to remove and don't run out of ink, but make sure you keep them sharpened.

I'm sure most of you will have tried the trick of programming yourself to wake up at a pre-arranged time, repeating the time over and over to yourself, banging your head on the pillow and all the other devices which people use. Amazingly, they work, and so does programming yourself to remember your dreams. When you get into bed and turn out the light, before you drift off, just tell yourself that you are going to remember your dreams when you wake up. Keep repeating this mental instruction for a couple of minutes, and try to picture yourself actually waking up, remembering your dream and writing it down. Sure enough, when you do waken the dream should be fresh in your memory. Turn on the light and immediately write down everything you can remember – colours, sounds, situations, emotions – don't worry about the order or about writing nonsense as it's the images which you have to record at this point. You'll make sense of them later.

I'm not suggesting that dream interpretation is in any way

a serious science, but by learning how to remember your dreams, writing down their content and looking at it in the cold, clear light of day you give yourself the opportunity of understanding the thought-processes which trigger the content of your dreams. You will be surprised at how frequently what you dream can provide you with pointers for solving specific problems. At its subconscious level your unfettered brain may be more likely to produce objective answers uncluttered with the ifs, buts and maybes of everyday life.

To rely on dream interpretation or to believe totally in the prophecy value of your dreams flies in the face of common sense. But to ignore your midnight excursions into madness altogether is extreme folly. If you've just dreamt the winner of tomorrow's 3.30, by all means have a bet on it, but don't mortgage the house.

Bad Dreams, Nightmares and Night Terrors

Bad dreams are those that wake you up in the night, although their content is not always that awful. Just as unpleasant experiences, rows, arguments, squabbles, failures, daily frustrations can cause stress and lead to insomnia, so when they are the subject of your dreams they may wake you and leave you in the state in which you started the night, namely worrying about the very event that occurred in your dreams. This is yet another strong argument for really persevering with relaxation techniques (see page 122). If this sort of problem is preying on your mind, try to blot it out at bedtime with some light reading or distracting and amusing entertainment on the radio or TV. Many late-night radio stations feature agony aunt phone-ins or problem programmes – I should know, I do them – and I get frequent letters from insomniac listeners who say that they fall asleep listening to everyone else's problems. Far from being upset by these letters, I am greatly encouraged by them, as it shows how being aware of the difficulties facing others enables us to forget our own, at least for long enough to fall asleep.

Going to bed with a full bladder or having drunk too much liquid late at night is not a good idea. The signals of the need to pass urine will intrude into your sleep and it is not uncommon both in older children and in adults for this to trigger the dream which becomes reality, a dream in which you are urinating and wake up to find that you have. This could be classified as a bad dream though it is a symptom of the strength of basic needs, including appetite and the need to empty the bowels. For this reason it's not a good idea to go to bed overhungry or on a very full stomach.

Sexual dreams are also sometimes categorised as being bad, an attitude with which I totally disagree. Even when sexual dreams are not being experienced during paradoxical sleep the penis is erect and there is an increased blood flow to the vagina, both signs of sexual arousal. Sexual dreams in men frequently end in ejaculation, in itself a physical and emotional release which engenders relaxation. As a result of either partner having sexual dreams couples may end up fondling each other or indeed wake to find themselves actively engaged in intercourse. Another frequent result of sexual fantasies while dreaming is masturbation, which tends to take place in both men and women during the half-sleep half-dozing period just before getting up.

There's nothing wrong with any of these situations. They are the subconscious at work, in line with Freud's theory of dreams as a route to self-indulgence. As long as self-indulgence is not one's code for conscious living, a little of it in the subconscious goes a long way to making your own private world a more relaxed place to live in.

Bad dreams are not the same as bad sleep and it's important that you are able to distinguish between a night disturbed by a sequence of bad dreams and a night of light, interrupted sleep which interferes with the proper balance between orthodox, paradoxical and deep sleep (see page 15). When your night is tormented by bad dreams there may be an overall reduction in the length of time during which you actually sleep, but the balance between the different sorts of sleep remains the same. This is because your dreams will tend to occur after a period of deep sleep and you will then wake at the beginning of light sleep and so remain in the proper rhythm. A long-term pattern of bad sleep – malsomnia – will certainly affect your state of mind and your ability to perform whilst awake. The occasional night disrupted by bad dreams does little harm and, in fact, can be extremely therapeutic, as these dreams help you to resolve and face up to fears, anxieties and problems which you make a very determined effort to avoid when you are awake.

Problems begin when the occasional disturbed night becomes a regular and frequent occurrence and you start to build up an accumulated sleep deficit over a period of time. In this situation you may well need some help in learning how to cope with your inability to face up to difficult practical or emotional situations, and to this end psychotherapy, hypnosis or counselling are all useful solutions. It's not hard for any individual to realise when they are suffering from malsomnia or bad dreams, and in this situation keeping your dream book up to date (see page 59) will give you a fascinating insight to the way in which your problem has arisen, and the roots from which it has grown.

Nightmares are a different story. They nearly always occur during paradoxical sleep and more often than not in one of the later phases in the sleep cycle. In all nightmares the scenario has one common thread – the inevitable harm, injury, damage or destruction inherent in the final outcome of these frightening dreams. As if the content of the dream were not frightening enough, the unpleasantness of the experience is dramatically reinforced by the apparent inability of the person woken or waking from a nightmare to move. This is typical of the paralysis-like immobility during paradoxical sleep. In a way they are rather like watching a complex and macabre TV soap opera in which all the characters are out to get you, the viewer. The locations are constantly changing, sometimes the screen is black and white, at other times it's full-blown technicolour and you may even view some scenes in bizarre and unreal hues. No matter how absurd the fantasy, how ludicrous the situation, how far removed from your own life the plot may be, these dreams are always vivid and terrifying.

Nightmares are common in children and seem to come in clusters at different stages in their development (see page 18), but for the rest of us they are a comparatively rare phenomenon, though few escape completely. It's not hard to pinpoint some cause for the occasional nightmare, but there is evidence to show that people who are very stressed and anxious are likely to suffer far more with nightmares than those lucky ones who are less stressed or who have learned to cope better with 20th-century living.

Just as the bad dream can leave you feeling tense and anxious, the nightmare leaves you feeling tense and very frightened. Again, if you seem to be getting nightmares on a regular basis, there is something going on inside your subconscious, or something which you are refusing to face up to consciously, and the puzzles need unravelling. If you think you fall into this category, do get some help, and get it sooner rather than later. The simple expedient of talking through your nightmares or discussing the problems in your life with a trained listener often results in increased self-awareness and a rapid reduction in the frequency of your nightmares. This is a boon for the sufferer but can also bring blessed respite to their sleeping partner, or more likely non-sleeping partner. As well as the inconvenience of being woken by a screaming, thrashing, nightmare-suffering incumbent of the same bed, the patient partner may also have to bear the brunt of physical assault as their hapless companion lashes out at the fantasy figures inhabiting their dream.

Night terrors are often confused with nightmares, but they are a totally different happening. Unlike the complex sequential stories of the nightmare, the night terror is a very simple and short dream which happens early in the night, soon after going into orthodox deep sleep. Night terrors are not the herald of some deeply disturbing psychological problem, but they may occur more frequently during periods of extreme stress and anxiety. They are far more common in children than in adults and show a very specific tendency to run in families. Typically a person in the grip of a night terror will be found bolt upright, wide-eyed and screaming. The episode may last anything from one to 15 minutes and is far more distressing for the watcher than the screamer, as there is hardly ever any memory of the event by the next morning. Night terrors in children are particularly hard on the parents (see page 145).

Commonly, night terrors go hand in hand with sleep-walking, and this, too, is more common in children, although it is estimated that around 2% of adults are occasionally affected. There are many myths surrounding sleep-walking – it's a sign of madness, it's dangerous to wake a sleep-walker, sleep-walkers never hurt themselves. These are all untrue: it's not a sign of madness; it is very difficult to wake a sleep-walker, it's best to try to lead him or her gently back to bed; as many as 25% of sleep-walkers are known to suffer some form of injury on their midnight wanderings. If you know you've got one in the house, it's worth making sure that you have a gate at the top of the stairs, that bedroom windows are securely shut or have protective bars and that you don't leave trailing electric cables, shin-high glass tables or fragile ornaments in their likely path.

There is great controversy about whether the sleep-walker is really asleep, awake or conscious. The answers to this question have considerable significance from a legal point of view, as it is not unknown for sleep-walkers to commit violent acts and the judicial outcome may well depend on establishing whether or not the somnambulist was aware of, or in control of, their actions. Recent research by Professor Crisp at St George's Hospital Medical School in London suggests that 'sleep-walkers are awake but in a state of mental dissociation that can sometimes lead to socially unacceptable but meaningful behaviour.'

Sleep-walking may immediately follow a night terror, and in the same way there is no memory of the nocturnal excursion the following morning, nor will there be any memory of the common ingredient of a sleep-walk, urination. This may or may not be performed in the appropriate room of the house.

Sleep-talking is frequently associated with sleep-walking, and likewise runs in families. It is not uncommon for the sleep-walker, particularly a young child, to be sleep-talking at the same time. Like the night terrors, when sleep-talking occurs on its own it tends to happen during orthodox sleep. The words are mostly gibberish and cause little or no disturbance to the talker, but can be nearly as bad an irritant to the listener as snoring, although on occasions rather more amusing. There are no known clinical effects of sleep-talking and the only social consequences depend on who says what to whom in whose bed.

Night terrors, sleep-walking and sleep-talking are not generally conditions which respond to any sort of treatment, nor is any needed if they are occasional occurrences. If they occur slightly more frequently at times of stress, this is understandable. If, on the other hand, any of them is becoming a serious problem either for the sleeper or those who are kept awake, then it is important to consider dietary factors and ways of dealing with stresses.

There is no doubt that anxiety will increase the frequency of all these happenings in the susceptible person, and if allowed to continue unchecked can, as so often with other sleep disorders, grow into a habit pattern that becomes difficult to reverse. Too much alcohol, too much caffeine, any stimulant drugs and, worst of all, the mixture of drugs and alcohol, will aggravate the problem. You may find that a small nip of alcohol helps you feel better during the daytime and gets you through the fears and anxieties that may go with your job or social responsibilities. As your body gradually eliminates the alcohol the anxiety returns and, if you've had a bit too much, you've got a headache to add to your other worries. Getting on to this merry-go-round is not merry at all, and will increase the frequency of nightmares, night terrors, sleep-walking and talking, whichever is appropriate to you.

Those of you who are cheese-lovers will be delighted to know that there is no evidence at all that eating cheese at bedtime causes nightmares. I am sure that this popular myth came from far too many passings of the port decanter round the table with the cheese in Victorian England, and as we've seen already it's certainly the alcohol that was to blame. Perhaps for fear of enraging the teetotal lobby it was felt better to continue enjoying the port and put the blame on the Stilton.

If you've been on long-term drug therapy using sleeping pills, tranquillisers, anti-depressants, in fact any of the behaviour-modifying drugs, trying to wean yourself off them will frequently produce a dramatic increase in all these nocturnal happenings, but that's a small price to pay for kicking the drug habit (see page 78).

Your best bet is to try some of the mild herbal calmatives (see page 89) and combine these with soothing herbal baths. In practice I have found these extremely effective. Children respond exceptionally well, as the surface area of their bodies is greater in proportion to their weight than adults, which allows a higher concentration of essential oils to be absorbed through the skin.

In general, dreams are a good thing, though you might find this difficult to believe if you've just woken up from your third horrific nightmare in a row. Don't be so pessimistic. Dreams give us all the opportunity to escape into a world of fantasy, to be king or queen for the day (or night), to be movie stars, opera singers, racing drivers, in fact to achieve things that in our waking hours seem beyond our wildest dreams.

When things go wrong, our dreams can be one of the earliest pointers, a prelude to depression, an indicator of stress, a messenger of anxiety. Get to know and understand your dreams, use them in a positive way and you will find them a rewarding, stimulating and therapeutic experience. Encourage your dreams, for they can be highly creative. History is full of examples of writers, poets and composers waking with the words or music bubbling out of them. Even scientists have put their dreams to good use. Einstein once suggested that the most creative scientists are those who have access to their dreams.

5

THE TYRANNY OF SLEEPING PILLS – HOW TO AVOID LIMPING THROUGH LIFE ON A CHEMICAL CRUTCH

'Sleep's the only medicine that gives us ease.'

Sophocles

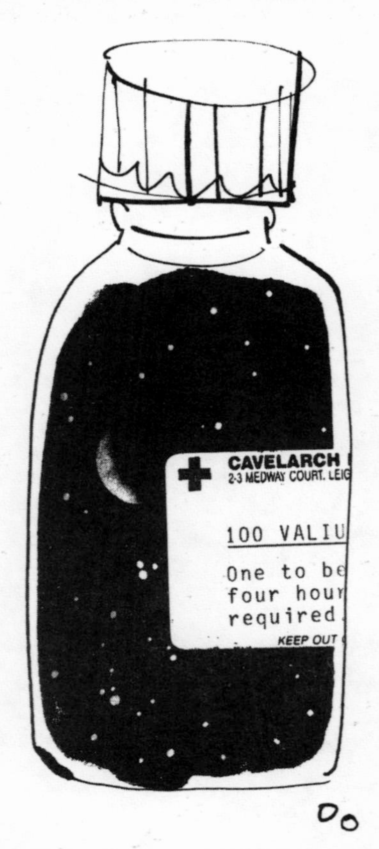

With one in every seven patients visiting their GP complaining of sleeping problems and one in four of all women middle-aged and onwards taking some form of medication for insomnia, it's obvious that the scale of this problem is huge. Throughout the UK several million people don't go to bed until they've taken some form of sedative or sleeping pill prescribed by their doctor, or a proprietary remedy which they've purchased over the counter. Some of these people will only take medication for short periods of time until the particular crisis which has caused their insomnia passes, but for the vast majority this pill-popping routine will continue for months or even years.

There is a vast army of people who are limping through life supported by a crutch of sleeping pills, sedatives and tranquillisers. And they limp. As we've seen, normal sleep falls into the two types, orthodox and paradoxical sleep, and virtually all sleeping drugs disrupt the normal patterns by suppressing paradoxical sleep. By taking these drugs you may get to sleep more easily, you may stay asleep longer, but the quality of your sleep may be seriously affected and the lingering effects of the drugs may be with you till well into the following day. They can impair judgement, concentration and physical ability, and this is just the beginning of your problem. There is no such thing as a totally safe drug. Any medicine which has an action may have a reaction, so the only remedy which has no side effect is one which has no effect either.

It's worth taking a hard look at the possible hazards of long-term drug therapy for chronic insomnia. It's worth knowing that 10% of all hospital admissions are the result of adverse reactions to prescribed medicines. It's worth knowing that for every doctor in practice in this country, the drug companies spend around £7,000 on advertising each year. It's certainly worth stopping before you take your next sleeping pill to wonder whether you really want or need to swallow it.

The idea of using drugs to help with sleep problems is not new. Our ancient forebears used magic mushrooms, hashish and the opium poppy long before Baron von Leibig created chloral hydrate and Adolf von Baeyer made the first barbiturates. Most of the modern drugs used for the treatment of sleep disorders are either anti-depressants, the minor and major tranquillisers or anti-histamines.

The first and by far the greatest risk of using sleeping pills is addiction or habituation. Since they interfere with the period of the sleep cycle in which dreams take place, it's very easy to get used to dreamless sleep. As soon as you try to stop taking the pills, sometimes after only very short periods, the sudden recurrence of dreams is likely to produce a few restless nights with a high probability of nightmares. It's quite natural to assume that sound sleep will elude you forever unless you take the pills. The truth is that it is those very pills that have caused the problem.

Coming off any form of sleeping pills must be a gradual process. Later in this chapter you will find a detailed programme to follow which will enable even the most hardened user of 'sleepers' to kick the habit over a period of two or three months.

Sedatives and Sleeping Pills

The function of these drugs is to modify your behaviour by their depressive effect on the normal activity of your brain. They can be used as sedatives to calm the nerves when prescribed in small doses, or as hypnotics which send you to sleep in larger doses. The most commonly prescribed of these drugs are:-

Chemical Name	**Brand Name**
alprazolam	Xanax
amylobarbitone	Amytal
butobartone	Soneryl
chloral hydrate	Noctec
chlordiazepoxide	Librium
chlormethiazole	Heminevrin

Chemical Name	Brand Name
chlormezanone	Trancopal
clobazam	Frisium
diazepam	Alupram, Atensine, Diazemuls, Evacalm, Solis, Stesomid, Tensium, Valium
dichloral phenazone	Welldorm
flurazepam	Dalmane, Paxane
lorazepam	Almazine, Ativan
nitrazepam	Mogadon, Nitrados, Noctesed, Remnos, Somnite, Surem, Unisomnia
oxazepam	Oxanid
prazepam	Centrax
promethazine	Phenergan
temazepam	Normison
triazolam	Halcion
triclofos sodium	Triclofos Elixir

None of these drugs mixes well with alcohol and the combination can have fatal consequences. Contrary to popular belief alcohol is not a stimulant but acts on the brain as a depressant; since sedative drugs work in the same way, the two together have a compounding effect. It is common for regular takers to build up a high level of tolerance to the drugs, which means that you have to take ever-increasing doses to achieve the same amount of sleep. The increased doses may cause your anxiety or depression to become worse, so the temptation is to take more medicine or more alcohol or both. Before you know it you are hooked in to a vicious circle which will inevitably lead to disaster.

Never leave your sleeping pills on the bedside table. It's the easiest thing in the world to wake in the night and pop another pill almost without realising what you are doing. The next time you wake in a now-befuddled state of mind you're likely to take yet more. So keep your pills in a locked bathroom cabinet and keep the key in a separate drawer.

The effect of these medicines on the elderly is another source of concern. Their bodies are not able to deal with drugs as efficiently as those of younger people and levels of these potent substances may build up in their bloodstream. This may make it more difficult for men, especially if they have prostate problems, to pass urine, and can also cause confusion, agitation and distress in both sexes. I am often appalled at the way in which elderly patients, when admitted to hospital and already confused by the unfamiliar surroundings, are routinely given sleeping pills. The chances are that these will only add to the patients' distress, and by the time they are discharged from the hospital they may well be hooked on them. A ward full of quiet, drugged, elderly patients (sadly the same applies to most other patients, too) may make life easier for an overworked and understaffed night-shift, but what does it do to the patients?

None of these drugs can be stopped suddenly without the risk of side effects. With some sensitive patients this can happen after they've been taking them for only two or three days and for most people it's probable after two or three weeks and inevitable after two or three months. Sensations of panic, irritability, sweating, tremors, hallucinations, terror, nausea, vomiting or loss of weight can all result from the withdrawal symptoms. Come off these drugs sensibly (see page 78).

Many of these drugs react extremely badly with other medicaments, so do tell any doctor prescribing further medication what you are already taking. Check with your pharmacist before using any over-the-counter medicines. It's also worth noting that some of these drugs can interfere with your body's absorption of vitamin D – which is essential for the body's efficient use of calcium and B_{12} – which is vital for the prevention of anaemia . . .?

None of these drugs should be taken during pregnancy or breast-feeding, nor should they be taken without specific advice from your doctor if you are suffering from heart or lung disease, kidney problems, liver disease, gout, digestive disorders or urinary conditions. Most of them are also not suitable for the treatment of hyperactive children.

Specific Problems with Sedatives and Sleeping Pills

Barbiturates like Amytal and Soneryl used to be the most widely prescribed of all sleeping pills. They are highly addictive and overdosing on barbiturates is extremely serious. In combination with alcohol an excessive intake of this type of medicine can easily result in death. They very quickly produce addiction and psychological habituation which is aggravated by the ease with which the body develops tolerance to this family of drugs. The tolerance means that larger and larger doses are required to produce sleep and, worryingly, regular users of barbiturates are often tempted to use alcohol to increase its effect. Barbiturates on their own cause intoxication very similar to drunkenness and when the two are mixed together the results can be appalling. Although the body will tolerate extremely large doses before sleep ensues, there is no tolerance to the lethal dose which can easily be taken in a vain attempt to get to sleep.

Happily these potent remedies are far less used today, but they should have no place in modern medicine as remedies for insomnia or anxiety, nor in daytime use as a sedative.

Chloral hydrate has less disruptive influence on paradoxical sleep but can cause stomach problems. Combined with alcohol its effects are legendary; this was the original recipe for that favourite of the thriller writer, the 'Mickey Finn'.

The Minor Tranquillisers – Benzodiazepines

The benzodiazepines are the group of drugs which includes Librium, Valium, Ativan, Xanax, Frisium, Tracopal and Tranzene. These are what was known as the minor tranqillisers or anti-anxiety drugs and are used as sedatives for the relief of anxiety, as anti-convulsants and muscle relaxants. In spite of the enormous adverse publicity surrounding the 'tranks', they are still heavily overprescribed.

It doesn't matter how small the dose is, all these tranquillisers have an adverse effect on the brain. They interfere with normal functioning of this vital organ and overall have a depressive effect. Small doses are used for their sedative and calming action, whilst larger doses will induce sleep.

Many members of this drug family commonly produce side effects including lightheadedness, sleepiness, poor co-ordination, an unsteady gait and sedation. Some people seem to be more sensitive to them than others and can suffer some side effects after just one dose, though these are more likely to occur after a period of time on the drugs. The effects on older patients may be severe.

There are few drugs which should be taken by breastfeeding mothers and hardly any which are safe during pregnancy, and this family of medicines is no exception. All the benzodiazepines affect the brain and in very long-term use they can be as bad as excessive alcohol consumption in this respect. Even short-term use can affect the way you perform complex functions which need co-ordination and mental agility. For this reason they are not suitable for drivers or for anyone working with machinery or in high risk situations – scaffolders, builders, firemen, window cleaners, dentists or surgeons!

Benzodiazepines are highly addictive and few people taking them regularly for more than four or five weeks are likely to be able to quit without problems. Going 'cold turkey' may produce severe withdrawal symptoms, panic attacks, tremors, excessive sweating, muscular aches and pains, anxiety, nausea, sensations of movement even when you're still, and worst of all, especially if this is the reason why you took them in the first place, insomnia.

There is a place for the use of these minor tranquillisers: for instance, since they are effective muscle relaxants they can help in the treatment of acute back pain. They may be of use immediately after a bereavement, to tide you over the initial shock and devastation, though in most situations it is more important to grieve naturally than to cover up the emotional upheaval. But they must all be treated with great caution, avoided wherever possible, and in any case they should never be used for more than seven days continuously.

The Anti-Depressants

This is a group of drugs developed for the relief of severe depression and in their proper place they are valuable. But as so often happens with powerful drugs, these too are being abused. For the busy doctor faced with too many patients in the waiting-room and too little time in the surgery, writing the prescription is the quickest way of ending the consultation. Patients suffering from serious depression need help in the form of counselling, psychotherapy or psychiatric treatment; there is no hope of solving their problems by sweeping the dirt under the carpet and covering up their symptoms with a bottle of pills.

One of the early signs of depression is often disruption of the normal sleeping patterns and drugs from this group are prescribed all too frequently for insomniac patients when doctors believe that depression is the underlying cause. The main medicines in this group are the monoamine oxidase inhibitors (MAOI), tricyclic and tetracyclic anti-depressants. These latter cyclic compounds are the most frequently prescribed for sleeplessness, and the commonest are:-

Chemical Name	**Brand Name**
amitriptyline	Domical, Elavil, Lentizol, Limbitrol, Triptafen, Tryptizol
butriptyline	Evadyne
clomipramine	Anafranil, Anafranil SR
desipramine	Pertofran
dothiepine	Prothiaden
imipramine	Praminil, Tofranil
mianserin	Bolvidon, Norval
nortriptyline	Allegron, Aventyl, Motival
trimipramine	Surmontil
viloxazine	Vivalan

The amitriptyline and trimipramine drugs are probably the most often prescribed for sleep disorders, but all the drugs can cause side effects, the most notable of which are urinary retention, constipation, dry mouth and an unpleasant taste, since they interfere with the production of saliva. All the tricyclic anti-depressants may carry extra risk when taken by people with urinary or prostate problems, liver or kidney disease, overactive thyroids, epilepsy, high blood pressure or glaucoma.

None of these drugs mixes well with alcohol and they may all react badly with local anaesthetics. The regular use of antacids and some diuretics can increase the effect of the anti-depressants, whilst the barbiturates and some other sleeping pills and oral contraceptives can reduce their effect. All the anti-depressants are likely to decrease the effectiveness of anti-histamines, asthma drugs, blood pressure drugs and some of the anti-convulsants. These drugs are generally not addictive but in view of their wide range of side effects they are not by any means a good long-term solution for insomnia.

L-Tryptophan – A warning that this may be dangerous

This is one of the essential amino acids, naturally present in many foods. It's important for the repair of protein tissues dissipated by the normal wear and tear of life and for the creation of new protein during growth. As long as there is sufficient vitamin B_6 (pyridoxine) in the diet, obtainable from brewers' yeast, liver, avocados, bananas, meat and poultry, tryptophan will be converted by the body into nicotinic acid and then into the chemical serotonin, which is a very powerful substance which affects the brain. Serotonin is linked directly to sleep patterns and actually induces sleepiness. The production of serotonin is also linked to daylight exposure (see page 50). It's recently been found that if there is a raised level of tryptophan in the bloodstream, more serotonin can get into the brain and help to promote feelings of sleepiness. For this reason it's probable that eating some form of carbohydrate at bedtime may be a help in the treatment of insomnia, as carbohydrates are a good source of tryptophan.

The use of tryptophan as a food supplement, available in high doses over the counter, and as a prescribed medicine (Pacitron and Optimax) for the treatment of insomnia and depression is now in serious question. A link has been established between preparations containing L-tryptophan and a potentially fatal condition known as eosinophilia-myalgia syndrome. Most of the cases have occurred in the USA, and 19 deaths and more than 1400 individual sufferers have been identified. Two cases associated with over-the-counter tryptophan preparations have already been reported in the UK, and it is probable that all products containing tryptophan will be withdrawn.

There is no danger whatsoever in eating foods containing natural tryptophan; the problem with the commercial products is believed to be contamination which occurs during the manufacturing process, though this is not yet absolutely certain. There are some similarities with the toxic oil syndrome epidemic which occurred in Spain in 1981 and was caused by adulteration of cooking oil. It is also possible that adverse reactions between tryptophan and benzodiazepines or tricyclic anti-depressants may be implicated.

This serves as a timely reminder that just because over-the-counter remedies or food supplements are 'natural', it does not necessarily mean that they are safe.

An End to Pill Dependence

Most people who take some form of pill every night in order to get to sleep would vehemently deny that they are drug addicts. Just like smokers, they say that they could give it up any time if they wanted. And unlike smokers they can justify this to themselves in the belief that without the pills they wouldn't sleep, and in order to function properly during the day they have to sleep. What they fail to realise is that all the drugs used to induce sleep have an adverse effect on brain function and on their ability to perform their normal daily tasks. They would almost certainly operate better without the drugs, with less sleep and without the 'hangover' effects that the medication produces. What's more, by following the advice throughout this book they should be able to re-educate their sleeping patterns and return to a life of trouble-free and pill-free nights.

Even if the drugs you are taking are not chemically addictive, they are certain to produce psychological dependence, especially when they are used for long periods of time. If you believe that you will never sleep again without a pill, then the chances are you won't. I have never forgotten the story told to me by one patient who for many years had collected her husband's prescription for barbiturates every month from the GP. When the family doctor retired, an enthusiastic and conscientious young man took his place, and within weeks had sent for her husband and told him he couldn't possibly allow the continuing use of these powerful drugs, and was going to replace them with much safer more modern tablets. The doctor then prescribed Mogadon and thought he'd done a good job.

Imagine his surprise when a few days later the irate wife appeared in his surgery complaining bitterly about the change which the doctor had made. The young medic was understandably more than a little upset by her attitude, but then crestfallen by her explanation. For years she had been opening the capsules of barbiturates, tipping the contents down the drain and refilling them with flour. How, she asked, could she possibly do that with tablets, and in any case her husband had slept perfectly well on half a teaspoon of flour every night.

Often the fact of taking the pill can have almost as much effect as what's in it. What you are going to do is to change your pill routine little by little over a period of weeks, or sometimes even months, until you get to the stage where you can manage on your own. Make sure that you are using the other sleep-inducing techniques which you will find in the rest of the book. Choose those which seem to suit you best and practice them regularly as a prelude to starting your own detox programme. If you have been a long-term user of sedatives, tranquillisers or sleeping pills, speak to your doctor before making any radical changes. He will certainly be delighted that you have made a positive effort to overcome your insomnia and he can help by giving you lower-dose medication which makes a planned reduction of your overall drug intake easier to achieve.

In order to re-establish your habitual sleeping pattern as it should be, you must pay particular heed to the section on good and bad habits (see page 25), and to all the information on sleeping patterns (see page 14). The time that you go to bed and get up is vitally important, as is the clockwork regularity of these two events. You need to build up a new and better set of reflex responses which correspond more closely with your natural rhythms than the reflexes which you have acquired over the years. In combination with all the other practical steps, this will lay the foundation for long-term solutions.

Few people can cope with throwing all their pills down the loo and saying never again. The best way is to take things step by step and to use as much time as necessary to achieve a successful outcome.

Step 1

Decide on the day that you are going to make changes that will set you on the path to drug-free sleep. Do not pick January 1st, as like most New Year's resolutions this one is bound to fall by the wayside. It's probably best to set a time about three or four weeks away for starting to reduce your medication.

Step 2

Once you've set the date, use the intervening time to improve your general state of health by reducing your alcohol intake, cutting down on your tea, coffee and chocolate consumption, and culminating in the seven-day diet plan (see page 36). Start taking some regular exercise, any sport that you enjoy, a regular cycle ride or even half an hour's walk each day.

Step 3

This is red letter day. By now you should be feeling a lot healthier and a little fitter. The very act of making a positive decision will probably mean that your sleep is already somewhat better. Arm yourself with any one of the natural calmatives like valerian, passiflora, hops, etc (see page 89), and proceed as follows.

Night 1 – take your normal dose of medication
Night 2 – take half the normal dose and the recommended dose of your alternative remedy
Night 3 – the normal dose
Night 4 – half the dose and alternative remedy
Night 5 – normal dose
Night 6 – half the dose and alternative remedy
Night 7 – half the dose and alternative remedy
Night 8 – normal dose
Night 9 – half the dose and alternative remedy
Night 10 – half the dose and alternative remedy
Night 11 – normal dose
Night 12 – half the dose and alternative remedy
Night 13 – half the dose and alternative remedy
Night 14 – half the dose and alternative remedy
Night 15 – normal dose
Nights 16, 17, 18 – half the dose and alternative remedy
Night 19 – normal dose
Nights 20, 21, 22, 23 – half the dose and alternative remedy
Night 24 – normal dose

Nights 25, 26, 27, 28 – half the dose and alternative remedy
Night 29 – normal dose
Nights 30, 31, 32, 33 – half the dose and alternative remedy
Night 34 – normal dose
Nights 35, 36, 37, 38, 39 – half the dose and alternative remedy
Night 40 – the last normal dose
Nights 41, 42, 43 – half the dose and alternative remedy
Night 44 – quarter of the dose and alternative remedy
Nights 45, 46, 47 – half the dose and alternative remedy
Night 48 – quarter of the dose and alternative remedy
Nights 49, 50 – half the dose and alternative remedy
Nights 51, 52, 53 – quarter of the dose and alternative remedy
Night 54 – half the dose and alternative remedy
Nights 55, 56, 57 – quarter of the dose and alternative remedy
Night 58 – the last half dose and alternative remedy
Night 59 – quarter of the dose and alternative remedy
Night 60 – alternative remedy only
Nights 61, 62, 63 – quarter of the dose and alternative remedy
Night 64 – alternative remedy only
Nights 65, 66 – quarter of the dose and alternative remedy
Night 67 – alternative only
Nights 68, 69 – quarter of the dose and alternative remedy
Nights 70, 71 – alternative only
Night 72 – quarter of the dose and alternative remedy
Nights 73, 74, 75 – alternative only
Night 76 – quarter of the dose and alternative remedy
Nights 77, 78, 79, 80 – alternative only
Night 81 – quarter of the dose and alternative remedy
Nights 82, 83, 84, 85, 86, 87 – alternative only
Night 88 – your last sleeping pill, quarter of the dose and alternative remedy
Night 89 – alternative only
Night 90 – half the alternative dose

It's taken you just three months to kick what may have been the habit of half a lifetime or more. It hasn't been easy. If you've had the occasional lapse it doesn't matter, but now you are gradually going to reduce the amount of alternative medication so that in the end you won't need anything at all. Carry on with the relaxation techniques you've been using, as they will help to tide you over difficult patches in your life, and we all have those from time to time. If you get really stuck go back to the alternative remedies as your first choice. Powerful sleeping pills and the other sedative and anti-anxiety drugs must be your last resort and then only for very short periods of 10–14 days at the absolute most.

Remember that going without sleep may seem like the end of the world, but it isn't. A few bad nights will not do you any real harm – no one ever died through lack of sleep, but thousands have died through taking too many pills. If during the programme you feel desperate, you're tossing and turning, throwing the bedclothes around, and hearing the clock chime every hour, get up and do something. Anything is better than lying in bed and worrying and everything is better than going back to the sleeping pills.

6

HERBS TO EAT, DRINK, TAKE, RUB ON, BATHE IN AND SMELL

'Anything green that grew out of the mould,
Was an excellent herb to our fathers of old.'

Rudyard Kipling

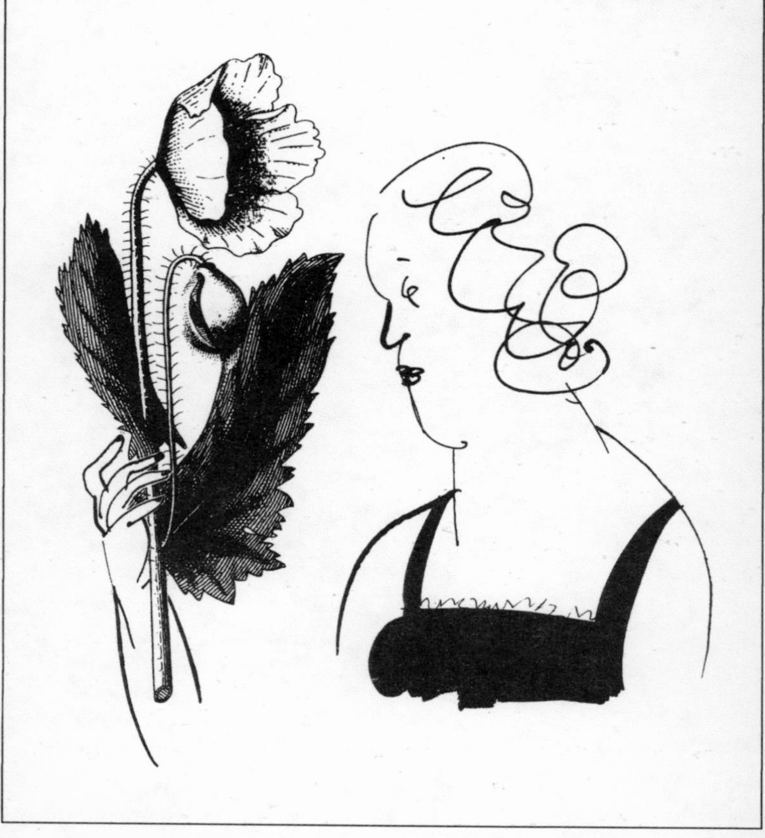

None of us can avoid those occasions when sleep defies even the most persistent somnolent. Some of us, most particularly the millions for whom this book is written, are chronically poor sleepers. We have already examined the pros and cons of the whole armoury of the drug industry and, now that you understand the inherent dangers that lurk inside every bottle of prescribed pills, you will naturally want to avoid them as far as possible. No, you are not expected to remain martyrs to your wakefulness, as there are a host of alternative remedies at your disposal. None of them addictive, none of them harmful, none of them on prescription, and many of them growing in your garden or in the hedgerows.

Since time began we have turned to the world of plants to provide relief from our aches and pains. Medicinal plants have even been found in Neanderthal graves. How did our ancestors know which ones to use? Certainly there must have been disasters, herbs which at best didn't work and at worst proved fatal. But there must also have been an instinctive understanding similar to that of animals. How else could it be possible that tribes as far apart as Fiji, Samoa, India, Trinidad and Vietnam all used the same preparation – hibiscus tea – to control fertility? What is even more surprising is that it probably worked, as the species of hibiscus they used has marked anti-oestrogen properties and helps to suppress ovulation just like the pill. Some 3,000 years before Christ, Chinese herbalists had written down their prescriptions; 1,000 years later the Babylonians carved their knowledge of plants on to tablets of stone – these even included specific sedatives. From the Ganges to the Nile remedies were traded.

Many new medicines were brought to England by the Romans. The first thing their physicians did when a new garrison was established was to plant a herb garden. The Welsh druids and the many monks around the country added to our knowledge and herbal medicine flourished right up to the early 20th century.

Then tragedy struck. Paul Ehrlich, the great Prussian biochemist, sounded the death knell of traditional herbal medicine with his 'magic bullets' concept of a pill for every ill. From this time on the pharmaceutical industry was on the rampage, dominating the whole drugs business. There's no doubt that many of the products of this industry have been a great boon to mankind, prolonging life, ensuring the survival of patients with diseases that in the past were almost inevitably fatal, and relieving pain. But sadly, the way in which they have taken over in the treatment of sickness has led to the rejection of herbal medicines, now so often dismissed as mumbo jumbo and misguided folklore. This in spite of the fact that many of the major 'new' drugs were derived from plants. Even now some 25% of all prescriptions contain at least one important ingredient from the herbal world. These components may be natural extracts or synthesised but they are vital parts of medicines like digoxin, atropine, vincristine, quinine, morphine, ephedrine and codeine, which are just a few of those in everyday use.

With a few notable exceptions like belladonna and other deadly poisons, most herbal remedies are both safe and effective, especially those available over the counter in the UK. Yet many doctors still regard plant remedies as little more than old wives' tales and continue to prescribe drugs where the gentler and nearly always cheapter use of herbs could well be far more appropriate as the first line of attack.

It's not surprising that the public has become uneasy about the overuse of powerful drugs, especially bearing in mind the side effects that many of them have. As a result more and more people are turning back to the traditional world of herbal medicines for the treatment of minor ailments and problems. Today there is ample scientific evidence to prove just how often all those old wives were right.

Evening primrose oil, for example, which provides relief from PMS, has been the subject of many studies which have shown that it also helps in the treatment of a wide range of other conditions, including multiple sclerosis, diabetes, heart and circulatory disease and even eczema, for which it is now available on prescription through the NHS.

Garlic, one of the most widely used of all medicinal plants, is now firmly established as a potent protector against heart disease. Large-scale clinical trials have shown that garlic tablets sharply reduced the death rate in a group of 400 patients who had already suffered one heart attack. It lowered cholesterol levels, reduced blood pressure, improved circulation and reduced the tendency to form blood clots.

One of the leading pioneers in the scientific testing of herbal medicines was a remarkable Swiss, Fred Pestalozzi. Nearly 40 years ago he was an engineer working in his home town of Zurich. His own experience of an incurable illness which was 'cured' by a herbal medicine led him to set up his own company in 1961 to produce the herbal medicine Bio-Strath. From the outset he was determined that his product would be a meeting of two worlds – the ancient world of traditional herbal wisdom and the modern world of scientific research.

Pestalozzi was intent on proving beyond doubt that his products were both safe and effective and he embarked on a research project on a scale never seen before in the herbal world. Scientists from universities and laboratories in England, Switzerland and Germany were persuaded to work on the experiments. At first they were all highly sceptical, but soon became enthusiastic as the results of their studies emerged.

This simple combination of herbs, yeast, orange juice and honey was shown to have far-reaching benefits as a general food supplement and tonic. Encouraged by the results, Pestalozzi went on to work with specific herbal medicines which resulted in a range of preparations including a combination of the Bio-Strath yeast with two of the traditional sedative herbs, valerian and passiflora. So effective is this product that, together with five others, it was granted a Medicines Licence by the British Government's Committee on Safety of Medicines. It was the first case of science proving folklore right.

A trip to any health food store or pharmacy will lead you to shelves of herbal medicines. Lots of these are of specific help in the relief of stress, anxiety, tension and insomnia. The traditional herbalist has always used extracts of hops, valerian, passiflora (passion flower), orange blossom, lime blossom, wild lettuce and skullcap. You will find these on sale in a variety of combinations, all of which are safe and non-addictive, but they do have a much milder action than prescribed sleeping pills. Be patient and persevere, it's worth the effort. Also be prepared to experiment a little and if after a couple of weeks' trial one particular formulation doesn't seem to be having much effect, try something different.

Even your local supermarket may have a wide selection of herbal teas and fresh herbs. You may think that these are just a way of avoiding caffeine or for use in cooking, but they often have the added bonus of powerful medicinal actions as well as their delicious flavours.

The folklore of herbs has always been a part of 'kitchen medicine', so later in the chapter is a list of the best recipes for a good night's sleep. Some of the ingredients will already be in your kitchen cupboards, but all of them are easily available.

A Goodnight Cuppa

In 1789 Sir John Hill, one of the great 18th-century herbalists, published *The Family Herbal*, subtitled 'An account of all those English plants which are remarkable for their virtues and of the drugs which are produced by vegetables of other countries'. The preface of his book could have been written 200 years later as his sentiments are just as appropriate today.

'When knowledge is perplexed with unintelligible terms, and the memory of the student confounded with a multiplicity of names; when the ignorant only, who have written concerning plants, have given themselves any trouble about their virtues; when physic is becoming entirely chymical, and a thousand lives are thrown away daily by these medicines, which might be saved by a better practice; it appeared a useful undertaking, to separate the necessary from the frivolous knowledge; and to lay before those who are inclined to do good to their distressed fellow-creatures, all that it is necessary for them to know of botany for that purpose, and that in the most familiar manner; and to add to this, what experience has confirmed of the many things written by others concerning their virtues.'

This remarkable book lists many herbs and plants to help the insomniac. Of wild lettuce Hill says, 'It eases the most violent pain in colics and other disorders and gently disposes the person to sleep. It has the good effect of a gentle opiate, and none of the bad ones of that violent medicine.' Of the lime tree he says, 'The flowers are good against giddiness of the head and all other lighter nervous disorders'.

The best way to use most of the helpful herbs is in the form of tea. Many herbal teas are available in a convenient tea-bag form today, but if you can't find the one you want, make your own. This is a simple procedure and nearly always involves the use of the aerial parts of the plant. That is, all the bits that grow above ground – leaves, stems, flowers – rather than the root. The easiest method is to use a proper infuser which keeps the plant material out of your cup, but you can use a teapot or a mug and pass the resulting brew through a fine tea strainer or a paper coffee filter to remove the bits.

As a general rule of thumb you will need one teaspoon of dried herb or two teaspoons of the fresh herb to a large cup or mug of boiling water. Cover the infusion and leave it to stand for at least ten minutes, strain, sweeten with a little honey if necessary – some of them are rather bitter – and sip slowly.

Amongst the traditional herbs which you should try as teas are: aniseed, balm, basil, borage, chamomile, fennel, hops, lemon verbena, lettuce, lime, marjoram, sage, savory, sweet cicely, valerian, vervain. All these work best if you have a cup about half an hour before bedtime.

If you really want to get the best out of herbs the answer is to grow your own. All of the following are easy to grow, in a herb garden. Many of them can also be grown in pots on a terrace, balcony, steps or even in window-boxes on the kitchen window-sill.

Here's all you need to know:

Balm: Otherwise known as Lemon Balm, this herb is equally helpful for calming nervous tension and the anxious, nervous indigestion that so often goes with it. Useful for over excited or anxious children too – in Spain it's considered a nursery cure-all. The leaves make a pleasant, soothing tea. It has a strong scent, but a much milder flavour, so is perfect as an addition to fruit salad, jellies, custard, or even to the more delicate soups. Best added towards the end of cooking as chopped leaves.

It is a hardy perennial which likes rich, moist soil and plenty of sun, but it will grow almost anywhere. The scent of the flowers is great for attracting bees – the ancient Greeks planted it for just this reason. Use the fresh leaves throughout the summer, but cut those you plan to dry just before flowering.

Basil: is both tonic and calming to the nervous system – a natural tranquilliser for the kind of frazzled nerves that lead to insomnia. If this is your problem, have a good *soupe au pistou* in the evening. Essential for any tomato dish; one of the best of all pasta sauces is 'pesto' made from basil, garlic, pine kernels and olive oil; add to soups, salads, fish and poultry; use with cooked vegetables like potatoes, courgettes, onions and beetroot. Never wash basil – the leaves turn black; wipe with a damp cloth and tear into small bits.

This is an annual in the UK as it really likes the southern sunshine. Grow in a well-drained pot in a sheltered, sunny spot. Bring into the house in September and keep on a sunny window-sill; you will have fresh leaves through the winter. They can be dried or frozen, but I prefer to use them to flavour a couple of bottles of olive oil.

Borage: the old herbalists used this pretty herb as an anti-depressant. Adding the leaves and flowers to wine was reputed to make people happy and carefree. It has a slightly cucumberish taste which makes the leaves ideal with fish, potato salad and cottage cheese. A sprig of leaves and flowers is the perfect complement to a glass of Pimms or cold red wine punch.

An annual which will self seed, can be grown in any soil, in a sunny position. Plant at least 2 ft (60 cm) from other plants. Use the young leaves during summer; the flowers can be picked fresh as needed, but for freezing or drying, gather them when just open.

Chamomile: insomnia, nervous indigestion and the jitters all respond to this magically calming herb, which makes one of the most pleasant of all herbal teas. Whenever ordinary tea or coffee is contra-indicated, this should be one of your first choices. It is one of the best indigestion cures, and has a good anti-inflammatory action which helps with joint problems and period pains.

A perennial which grows just about anywhere and is ideal for pots or troughs as well as gardens. Use the fresh flowers for your tea, and pick them to dry when they are in full bloom.

Fennel: the seeds and the feathery fronds are equally effective aids to digestion. Tea made from the crushed, dried seeds is a remedy for gas, colic or stomach cramps. A similar, but stronger flavour than dill. The perfect herb for oily fish like herring and mackerel, which should be grilled on sprigs of it. The chopped fronds can be sprinkled on salads and vegetables, and add the seeds to the liquid used for poached fish.

A hardy perennial which does well in the garden or pots, but needs some sun. The fresh fronds are good for freezing but not for drying.

Lemon Verbena: a much stronger flavour than lemon balm and longer lasting, this beautiful herb makes a delicious and strongly sedative tea.

A deciduous perennial which may suffer in severe winters. It will do best in a sheltered spot, against a south-facing wall and in well-drained soil. It can grow to about 8 ft (2.5 m), but a pot will restrict the growth, and allow the plant to be taken in during bad winters.

Use the fresh leaves up to late September, but ones for drying should be gathered just before flowering.

Marjoram (or Oregano): the volatile oil of this aromatic herb is powerfully sedative and, in fact, it is one of the great calmers. Use it for nerves and indigestion. It is a good remedy for chest infections, so eat lots of it during the winter months. Add it to salads, or at the end of cooking to soups, meat dishes, poultry, winter stews, vegetables and, sparingly, to cheese dishes. The wonderful aromas of Italian cooking come mainly from the wild marjoram or oregano. Wherever pizza is in the oven, or tomatoes in the pan, oregano is there too.

All the marjorams are easy to grow, and will do well in pots. Sow the seeds in April, or divide established plants in late summer. They prefer light, well-drained soil and sunshine. Pick fresh shoots from spring to autumn. Sweet marjoram is the only variety that dries well, and you should pick whole shoots with leaves and flowers.

Sage: a powerful antiseptic and healer (try it as a gargle for sore throats). It also acts as a stimulant to the central nervous system, making it a valuable tonic for convalescence, or for those suffering from stress or nervous exaustion. This herb is a good aid to digestion, particularly of fatty foods, so using it in the stuffing of roast meats and poultry is a sound idea.

The slightly bitter taste goes well with liver, duck, goose, pork, sausages and stews. Except with fried calves liver, when whole leaves are used, the leaves should be chopped.

These hardy, evergreen shrubs grow well in pots or in light, well-drained soil. They like the sun.

Pick the leaves fresh when needed, but for drying they need to be gathered just before the bush flowers.

Savory: its German name means 'bean-herb' since it eases the digestion of even this challenging food, and benefits the entire digestive tract. It has an antiseptic action on the gut and its aphrodisiac powers are legendary – but no doubt exaggerated. Flatulence is a common cause of insomnia – both for the sufferer and his or her partner!

The slightly peppery taste mixes well with other herbs, and is good for all bean dishes, in soups, marinades, with fish, poultry, game and pork.

The two varieties are winter and summer savory. The former has a stronger taste, so use sparingly. They both do well in pots, and like well-drained soil and sunshine. Use fresh leaves and pick shoots for drying before the plants flower.

Sweet Cicely: this favourite of the old herbalists is said to be relaxing, a good digestive aid, helpful for flatulence and a good expectorant.

The leaves and young fruits may be chewed – they have a slight aniseed flavour. The chopped leaves are good in soups and salads, also with all the root vegetables. A good use of this herb is to add sprigs of the fresh plant to sour fruits like rhubarb, plums, damsons, berries and currants; this sweetens the fruit and reduces the quantity of sugar needed in cooking. The chopped leaves can be sprinkled on to fresh strawberries or gooseberries.

It will grow anywhere, but does best in damp soil and half shade. The leaves freeze, but are not suitable for drying.

Of course, none of these safe herbal products has the same powerful effect as prescribed drugs. They are gentler, they take longer to work, and you need to persevere with them. On the other hand, they are easy to stop when you no longer need them, they have no side effects, and they are simple to use. Some of the remedies are best taken in medicinal doses or tablets, some can be used as teas, some can be rubbed on as oils, some can be added to your bath, and some work if you just inhale their wonderful aromatic smells. You might find any one, or any combination, the ideal solution to your problems, so have a go and keep experimenting until you find the mixture of therapies that suits you best. Even if you don't pick the right combination first time off, it's great fun trying – especially the ones that are massaged in!

The Magic of Massage

Almost everywhere else in the world massage is regarded as one of the great and beneficial forms of therapy. In England – where we seem to have problems touching ourselves, let alone other people – this wonderful form of treatment has always been endowed with a taint of smuttiness and sexuality. Of course massage can be sexy if that's what you want, but there is a world of difference between sexuality and sensuality and the best of massage is indeed sensual. It stimulates the senses because it is a touch therapy and, when it is combined with the use of perfumed essential oils, the effects can be greatly enhanced.

Even the most stoic of Englishmen complete with stiff upper lip, bull neck, military bearing and all the other stereotyped attributes, can learn to enjoy and benefit from a good massage. It's not always easy to persuade him to try it in the first place, but once you have there's no stopping him. We all have the ability to massage and there's no need to go on special courses or to undertake any particular training, unless you plan to take it up professionally. There are, however, lots of excellent short courses for those who want to learn the basics of massage to use with family and friends, and there are excellent books which give you the outline. But every mother already knows how to do it. You rub your baby's back to bring up the wind, you soothe away the pain of bumps, all without anyone to teach you how. Touching is instinctive and healing.

Tension, stress and anxiety are common factors in virtually all insomniacs. Overcoming these with massage is one of the first steps to better sleep. Unfortunately this is not one that you can take for yourself, you need a willing partner or a good friend, but mastering the simple art of massage will do wonders for both the insomniac and the relationship.

One of the most popular modern forms of therapy, and also one of the most ancient of all the healing arts, is aromatherapy, the combination of massage with aromatic plant oils. Not only does the recipient have all the benefits of massage, but added to these are the bonuses of the medicinal activity of the essential plant oils. The actual smells are beneficial in themselves, as they can create feelings of calm, peace, relaxation, comfort and de-stressing. Although people assume that the skin lets sweat out and nothing in, this is wrong. The chemicals in essential oils are very easily absorbed by the skin, and recent scientific studies have shown how quickly these substances appear in exhaled breath after being rubbed on to the surface of the body or added to a warm bath in which the subject is immersed.

First let's look at some of the aromatherapy oils and how they should be used. When doing any sort of massage it's important to have a good lubricating medium between your hands and the skin. Not only does this make the massage more comfortable for the subject, but it is more comfortable for the masseur's hands too. Some people use talcum powder, but this is not an option which I would ever recommend as it doesn't form a good link and can have irritant effects on the skin. As we are going to be adding essential aromatic oils to our massage oil it is important that the base oil should have very little smell of its own. You can use almost any oil for massage but the best are pure cold-pressed oils like sunflower seed or grape seed. These are both light, non-greasy and very well absorbed by the skin. They have the added benefit of not being too expensive. Most aromatherapists add a little wheatgerm oil to their basic mix as its very high content of vitamin E helps to preserve the other oils. The importance of this basic oil is that it acts as a carrier and enables you to apply the expensive and highly potent essential oils in an effective way to the skin.

Ideally you should prepare fairly small quantities of your basic oil; then you can experiment with the aromatherapy additions till you find the mixture that suits you best, and of course you can alter your prescription to fit particular needs. You must use a glass bottle with a tightly fitting screw top or ground glass stopper; the bottle should ideally be coloured to keep out the light. This helps to preserve your oils in their best condition. Every woman knows about the benefits of avocado oil to the skin, it's a very effective carrier and helps to encourage other essential oils to penetrate the skin. For this reason I normally add a little (it's expensive) to the basic recipe as follows.

You will need a 100cc coloured glass bottle with tight-fitting stopper into which you put:

10cc avocado oil
10cc wheatgerm oil
80cc grape seed oil

(100cc is slightly less than 4 fluid ounces)

You are now ready to add your essential oils. Good essential oils are expensive but you need to use very little of them. Don't be tempted to buy the cheaper blends of essential oils as these may contain alcohol and other adulterants which help to enhance their fragrance. Choose good quality, pure, unblended, essential oils and don't be tempted to be pennywise and pound foolish by going for the cheaper options. A good source is Rakan Distribution Ltd, 35 Goldsworth Rd, Woking, Surrey. You are bound to make a few mistakes to start with, and it is very much a question of trial and error to find the blend of essential oils which suits you best when added to your basic massage mixture.

In order to avoid ending up with a 100cc bottle which smells revolting and will keep your friends away from you for weeks, the best solution is to pour a little of your basic mixture into an egg cup and add literally one or two drops of essential oils. Use this as a way of finding a mixture of appropriate oils which creates a fragrance you like. Keep a careful note of the oils which you add and when you come to your final choice you can then make up your big bottle for regular use.

The mixtures which I have found most effective are:

For general insomnia: 2 drops of chamomile, 3 drops of juniper, 3 drops of marjoram.

For stress with associated insomnia: 2 drops of chamomile, 5 drops of melissa, 3 drops of rose.

For headaches: 6 drops of sage, 3 drops of rose, 5 drops of melissa, 5 drops of lavender.

If you are feeling nervy: 5 drops of bergamot, 3 of neroli, 3 of sandalwood, 5 of marjoram.

To pep you up after a bad night's sleep: 8 drops of fennel, 3 drops of sage, 4 drops of rosemary, 1 drop of juniper.

If it's the cough that's keeping you awake: try 6 drops of hyssop, 7 drops of eucalyptus and 2 drops of sandalwood.

For a stuffy nose or a cold: relieve the congestion with 5 drops of basil, 3 drops of eucalyptus, 3 drops of peppermint.

And if what you need is an all purpose oil to soothe those aching muscles which keep you awake after a day in the garden or a workout in the gym, try 6 drops of rosemary, 4 drops of sage, and 5 drops of eucalyptus.

Any of these mixtures can be added to your basic massage oil; allow 10 drops of the mixed essential oils to half an egg cup of massage oil to make up your trial samples. The mixtures can also be used with great benefits in your bath. Ten to 15 drops in the average-sized bath is all you need – and, of course, the time for a good wallow.

Once you find mixtures that you like, you can keep them in small dropper bottles ready to add to the bath or your massage oil, and if you are making up a larger quantity of oil you can substitute the drop measures given above with ccs and add to one litre of basic massage oil.

A few words about the practical applications of massage. It's important that both the donor and the recipient are comfortable. It's no good trying to massage your partner on the lower level of a bunk bed or on a cold floor near the draughty French windows. You need warmth, peace and quiet and some soothing music; take the phone off the hook. It's a good idea to have a few large towels handy so that you can keep the bits that you're not actually working on covered and warm, and cover them again immediately after the massage. Don't confine the treatment to bed-time, as although this is the ideal moment to help the insomniac, the occasional massage at other times of the day will help to reduce levels of stress and muscle tension.

The most common site of physical tension which is the result of emotional stress, or occupational and postural stress like typing, word-processing, sitting at a switchboard or check-out counter, leaning over a drawing-board, doing the ironing, is the neck. The large muscles which support the head and those which form the shoulders can knot up to the extent of feeling like planks of wood to the touch. These contracted muscles act like a giant spring, squeezing the small vertebrae in the neck together, putting pressure on the nerves, which causes pain, which causes more muscle contraction, which causes more pain. The result – headache, neckache, face ache, earache, jaw ache, shoulder ache, insomnia.

This is the point at which even the most amateur of masseurs can bring unbelievable relief. With problems in this area it is often easier to have the patient sitting rather than lying, as this avoids the additional problem of turning the head to one side or the other. Put a chair about 18 in (45 cm) away from the kitchen- or dining-table. Place a thick cushion on the table and position your subject so that they are sitting comfortably on the chair, feet slightly apart and flat on the floor, leaning foward with their elbows on the cushion and fingers together, palms down. With the forehead resting on the hands fairly close to the edge of the cushion and table, it's easy to breathe without turning the head to the side.

Stand directly behind your subject, or, if you find it more comfortable, to one side or the other. Warm your bottle of massage oil in a bowl of hot water, pour a little into the palm of one hand, rub the hands together and gently smooth the oil over the back of the subject's neck, upper back and shoulders. From this point do not break your contact with the subject's skin until you have finished the massage. Even if you are moving from one side of the chair to the other, always keep one hand touching the skin. Each time you make and break that contact, you interrupt the process of relaxation.

Having applied the oil, move both hands up to the top of the shoulders, so that your fingers just curl comfortably over the ridge of muscle that goes from the base of the neck to the point of the shoulder, and your thumbs will be pointing towards the bottom of the spine. Start a gentle kneading motion moving your thumbs from the back of the shoulder up each side of the bones in the neck, while squeezing your fingers towards the thumb and the palm of the hand. You should then end up with your thumbs at the base of the skull, and your fingers around the side of the neck. Slide the hands down to the starting position and repeat. Never poke or prod with the tips of your fingers – this does not feel nice or relaxing. All the movements of your hands and fingers should be rhythmic, slow and applied with firm but comfortable pressure. The pads of the fingers and thumbs, the soft fleshy part around the ball of your thumb and the whole palm of the hand are the bits that make the best contact.

Carry on massaging the neck and upper shoulders for three or four minutes, then move your hands further down the back so that your thumbs are on either side of the spine 2in (5cm) below the shoulder blades, and your fingers are fanned out across the shoulder blade on each side.

Move the thumbs up on either side of the spine and when you get to the top of the shoulder blade, slide them out towards the outside tip of the shoulder, keeping your fingers quite rigid so that they push a gentle ripple of flesh as they go. When you get to the tip of the shoulder, slide the hands down the outside of the ribs to the bottom of the rib cage, then into the centre, and start again. Continue this for at least five or six minutes.

Now it's time to get to the head. Slide the hands up the centre of the back, up the neck, over the side of the face to the temples, and gently rub in a circular motion moving your hands slowly forward as far as they can go before hitting the cushion, and then back again over the temple, over the top of the ears and down behind the ears. After a few minutes of this treatment you can gently lift your subject's head while you stand directly behind the chair and let the head rest on your chest. Then slide the fingers forwards again until they meet in the middle of the forehead. At this point you can start to massage very gently using the tips of your fingers in this case, with outward strokes from the centre of the forehead, over the eye to the temple. You can then move to the bridge of the nose and apply the lightest of pressure to the sinus areas under the eye and around the eye socket. After three or four minutes of this, gently ease the head forward, back on to the cushion, move to one side of the chair, not forgetting to maintain contact with the skin, and do a few final minutes' work on the neck.

From this position use one hand to support the head and stop it rolling from side to side and use the other with your thumb on the side of the neck nearest to you, and your fingers on the opposite side, and work your way in gentle circular movements up and down the muscles on the side of the neck.

What you will find surprising is that as you get used to the technique and stop worrying about whether you're doing it right or not, you will feel as relaxed as the result of giving the massage as your fortunate friend who's been lucky enough to receive it.

Other common areas that suffer from the stresses of everyday life are the lower back and the muscles of the buttocks, and these are both rewarding to massage as, with very little practice, your fingers will be able to feel the tension dissolving out of the muscles as you work on them. To work on this region your subject must be lying face down, but most beds are far too soft and standing at the side of the bed will almost certainly mean you end up with backache as well. A duvet, a couple of thick blankets or a foam mattress on the floor is the next best thing to a proper massage table. You can kneel beside it, at either end of it, or astride your patient which enables you to work fairly comfortably.

Once again, warm up your oil, pour some into a cupped palm, rub the hands together and spread it over the whole back and buttock area. Start with your thumbs just over the dimples on either side of the base of the spine and your fingers spread over the tops of the buttocks. Using your body weight to apply the pressure, lean gently forwards and slide your thumbs along the big muscles on either side of the spine with your fingers spread over the outside of the trunk and pointing slightly forwards. When you get to the lower part of the ribcage, release the pressure a little and slide the hands back to the starting position. After a dozen or so strokes, start moving the thumbs outwards as you get to the middle part of the back, move the whole hand round the ribcage and slide back towards the hip bones squeezing gently. When you reach the pelvis slide the hands back into the middle and repeat this a few more times. Then moving to one side of your subject, place your thumb parallel with the spine on the side of the spine furthest from you and pointing towards the head, the fingers curling round the flank. Using the other hand resting on top of the hand in contact with the muscles to apply the pressure, push your thumb straight across the muscle towards the floor. At the same time cup your fingers so that you gather a roll of muscle into the palm of your hand. When you reach as far as you can round the body, release the thumb pressure, keeping the fingers in contact with the skin, pull the hand back to the middle again and move it up about 1 in (2.5 cm). Repeat this movement until you have worked your way up to the shoulder blade, then work your way gradually down again. Repeat this sequence two or three times, then change sides and do it all again.

Finally, attack the buttocks. These are big powerful muscles and need a fair amount of muscle power from the masseur if you're going to make any impression on them. Treat the buttock muscles as you would a lump of dough on your pastry board. Knead them, squeeze them, roll them, and if you're fairly small and your subject fairly large and muscular you can even use the point of your elbow as an instrument and just lean your body weight into the muscles and move the elbow in small circles.

Hands and feet should never be forgotten. Massaging these is incredibly soothing but beware the ticklish foot. You must apply firm direct pressure and be very positive about what you are doing. One of the most comfortable ways of dealing with feet is to sit in a chair and have your subject lying on the floor and placing one foot at a time in your lap. Apply the oil in the usual way and then, using both hands, start with your thumbs on the sole of the foot pointing towards the toes, and fingers curled round the arch. Apply pressure firmly with the thumbs and the fingers at the same time in a pincer-like movement working the thumbs in small circles up and down the sole of the foot. Massage each toe individually, use thumb and forefinger on either side of the Achilles tendon, but don't squeeze too hard as this can be very tender, and work your hands in a kneading motion up the back of the calf. Return to the starting position with hands on the foot and move the hands in opposite directions so that you are mobilising and relaxing the joints of the foot. You can end a foot massage with a warm footbath, using any of the essential oil mixtures.

Do the same treatment to the hands and fingers, and massage the arms by holding the subject's hand in one of yours and moving the other hand up and down the arm in a fairly light but rhythmic stroking movement.

The combination of massage and the relaxing essential oils is a true passport to the Land of Nod. Don't expect it to produce instant miracle cures for months or even years of insomnia, but it will quickly help to establish better patterns of getting to sleep, and this is a major step in the right direction. As an added bonus, regular massage helps to prevent muscles from becoming fibrous and rigid, and at the same time stimulates and improves the circulation. It is almost impossible to do any harm or damage with sensible and gentle massage; however, there are some contra-indications. Never use massage on anyone who has severe skin problems, especially if there are open or infected sores and rashes. Don't massage anybody who has recently suffered from any form of thrombosis, and never massage any area of the body which is obviously red, hot and inflamed.

Don't sniff at smells

Most people are not consciously aware of what a powerful effect smells can have on them. We all recognise nice smells and nasty smells, but through the gradual process of evolution our sense of smell has become less important as a means of survival, so we have tended to minimise its value and its importance. Smells can be just about the most evocative of all the stimulants to our sensory perceptions. Just think how the faintest whiff of perfume can remind you of a long dead grandmother, a first girlfriend or a frightening teacher. The scent of a particular pine tree can bring back memories of distant holidays. A waft of cooking smells can transport you instantly back to your mother's kitchen. So powerful is the impact of smell that psychologists are now using bottled, artificial smells of gas works, steam trains and the seaside to treat elderly patients with depression. These amazing combinations remind them of their youth and of happier times and this particular form of therapy is proving highly successful.

The perfumed boudoir has always been a favourite of the romantic novelist, and not without reason. Cleopatra understood the power of fragrance, so why not take a leaf out of her book and create an ideal ambience for restful sleep in your bedroom?

Many of the aromatic herbs retain their essential oils when they are dried. Gentle warmth will release these oils into the atmosphere, and for this reason herb pillows are an excellent aid to better sleep. Body heat is enough to release the oils and the wonderful fragrances which they carry. You can buy herb pillows, but it is more fun to make your own and you can mix the herbs so that the resulting perfume is to your taste. A hop-filled pillow is one of the most effective but in fact the smell of hops is not that pleasant. Combine them with lavender, rose petals, cloves, lemon balm, verbena, rosemary, thyme, and most especially woodruff, which is a great aid to sleeping and smells wonderful.

A large bowl of pot pourri in the bedroom using a selection from the same herbs is a must. It's really worth the trouble of making up your own unique mixture. It will give your bedroom a delicate hint of a fragrance which will be all your own and will pervade the room with soporific scents. Use the same mixture to fill small bags which you can place amongst your nighties or pyjamas so that they too will give off the soothing vapours.

A last hint about herbs. Some people find that it is easier to sleep with a tiny glimmer of light in the bedroom. You can kill two birds with one stone by using one of the small pottery candle holders which at the same time serves as a means of heating up essential oils. One of the most soothing of all is orange blossom, but don't forget to fill the top of your dispenser with water before adding four or five drops of oil. Light your night light and go to bed. The delicate smell of orange blossom will pervade your room and help to keep your senses dulled till morning.

7

FAT PEOPLE SLEEP BETTER: DIETERS LOSE SLEEP AS WELL AS WEIGHT

'A good Kitchen is a good Apothicaries shop'

William Bullein, 1576

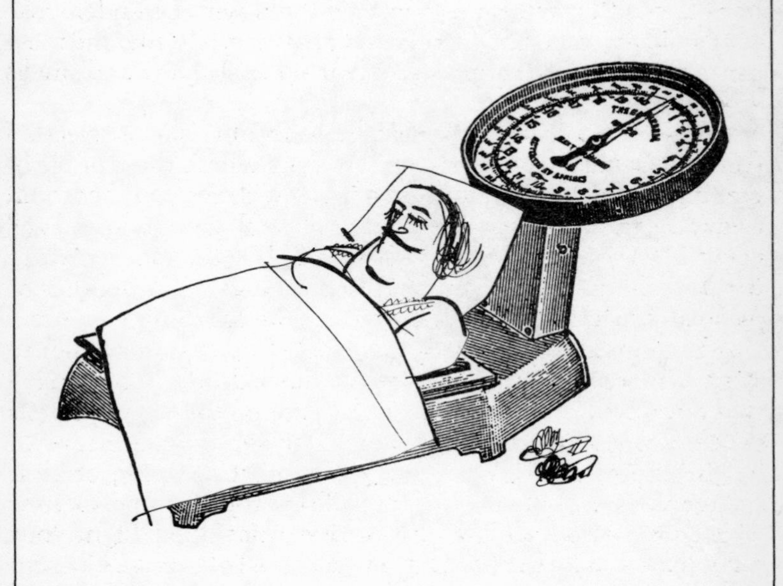

Without doubt, one of the most commonly held beliefs about fat and thin people is that the first are happy and the second less so. This conception is enshrined in our literary heritage. You only need to compare the ebullient, jolly, roly-poly Mr Pickwick with the lean and hungry Cassius. Both Dickens and Shakespeare understood this difference and exploited it widely: consider Scrooge and Falstaff, Uriah Heep and Mistress Quickly. Writers, playwrights and even – in more modern times – the creators of television series have drawn on this fundamental difference in order to highlight two extremes of the human condition.

Despite the efforts of the slimming lobby to persuade us that all overweight people are, in truth, desperately miserable and unhappy thinnies struggling to get out of their fat shells, and the tireless attempts of the advertising industry to project all that is good, beautiful, desirable and aspirational as thin, Shakespeare and Dickens got it just about right.

We have seen already that anxious people sleep less well than happy ones. We also know that happy people have better appetites and a better ability to absorb food than those suffering from anxiety. The happy bunch inevitably have a tendency to gain weight, whilst the unhappy are more likely to lose it, sometimes even unwittingly.

As always, there are exceptions that prove the rule, and occasionally the response to anxiety, stress and unhappiness is 'comfort eating' and subsequent weight gain. This is far less common, though.

The scientific link between weight and sleep was first described in a paper published in the British Medical Journal in 1976 by Professor Arthur Crisp. He and his researchers conducted a random survey of 1,000 men and women. They were all weighed and asked a selection of questions with the object of determining how they felt about themselves, specifically in relation to anxiety and depression. The end result showed that the overweight members of the group were more satisfied with life and generally of a happier disposition than their thinner counterparts. Happiness is equated with sleeping well, whereas anxiety and depression almost inevitably lead to sleep of less quality and more disruption. Overall, the overweight slept for longer and they enjoyed proportionately more paradoxical sleep (see page 10). It is during this phase of sleep that the greatest degree of muscular relaxation occurs – waking from paradoxical sleep frequently results in momentary sensations of paralysis – and more paradoxical sleep means renewed energy the following day.

There is no denying that the thin, over-anxious, tense person is far more likely to suffer from sleep problems. Overcoming the root cause of the anxiety and depression (see page 121) is a prerequisite to improving sleep habits. These mental anxiety states are frequently the result of an inability to cope with the demands of life, but appropriate psychotherapy will usually resolve the problem in time.

Faulty eating habits, on the other hand, can produce far more intractable problems and this is even more so in self-inflicted nutritional deprivation. There is currently a vogue for a whole range of extreme dietary regimes, none of them healthy, none of them with any basis in sound scientific fact and none of them to be recommended. Whether an individual takes it upon himself to follow some absurd guru, or whether dietary changes are recommended directly by any one of the myriad of alternative health practitioners, the end result will be the same.

It is rare to see obvious clinical signs of malnutrition in this country, save in the case of anorexia nervosa, but more of that later. What is disturbingly common is the incidence of 'sub-clinical' malnutrition – that is, the accumulated deficit in essential nutrients which is not enough to cause scurvy, ricketts or beri-beri, but is sufficient to interfere with the efficient workings of the body's biological machine. This disturbance of function almost invariably leads to disturbance of sleep.

Why do people go on to these ridiculous diets? Sometimes out of pure vanity, sometimes through social pressures imposed by peers, occupational demands or even family interference. They may have been told they suffer from food allergies; they may have been prescribed an outrageous diet for the treatment of candida (a condition which, though currently fashionable in alternative medicine circles, has yet to be supported by a shred of medical evidence in the majority of cases).

Beware the so-called nutritionists who are not complementary practitioners, nor alternative practioners, they're not even fringe practitioners. What they are is beyond the fringe – most of them with worthless diplomas graciously bestowed, in return for large amounts of money, by establishments whose prime objective is to train salesmen and women in the art of foisting their own particular products on to an unsuspecting public in the guise of nutritional counselling. These people play on the emotions of an unsuspecting public. One recently reported case was that of a teenage boy who developed epilepsy. The parents, not wishing to accept this diagnosis, grasped at the straw of beyond-the-fringe medicine, and consulted a practitioner who pronounced their son to have food allergies. He was put on a very restricted diet which produced no improvement. They took him to another practitioner, who removed even more foods from his diet. By the time he'd been to the third charlatan he was living exclusively on only five different foods. When admitted to hospital he was suffering from severe scurvy and hours from death. And, of course, he still had his epilepsy.

This is an extreme story, but a warning to those who decide to follow ridiculous dietary regimes based on bogus diagnoses and prescribed by totally unqualified and irresponsible practitioners. Just because you are faced with a man in a white coat with a row of glossy diplomas (mostly not worth the paper they're printed on), don't suspend your own powers of critical judgement or commonsense.

Anorexia nervosa is a completely different matter and needs intensive psychiatric intervention and psychological counselling. As in all cases of nutritional deprivation, sleep patterns are affected early on. It is well documented that as dieters lose weight, they sleep less. This pattern is not so much a reflection of the quantity of food being eaten, but of the total body weight.

Studies on anorexics show that at the beginning of treatment, although they were being fed a good diet but were still very thin, they tended to fall asleep normally but wake up very early and were unable to get back to sleep. As their weight increased, the length of time they stayed asleep gradually increased and by the time their weight was normal, so was their sleep.

The moral is clear: if you are already suffering from insomnia, don't go on a weight-loss diet. If you are underweight, putting on a few pounds will help to improve your sleep. If you are overweight with a sleep problem, this is not the time to think about reducing, unless of course there are serious medical reasons why you should – heart disease, severe breathing problems or if you're awaiting surgery.

Severe obesity, on the other hand, can also interfere with your sleep. It adversely affects breathing, increases the likelihood of disruptive snoring and may lead to sleep apnoea (see page 114). Carrying excessive weight encourages degenerative arthritic changes in the weight-bearing joints, spine, hips, knees and ankles. Arthritis is extremely painful, and pain disrupts sleep. If you do need to lose weight, make sure you follow a sensible dietary regime (see page 36). Do not use very low calorie meal replacements, mono-diets or any extreme eating plan which does not supply you with a full spectrum of food sources or sufficient calories to enable you to carry on with your normal daily activities.

Never go to bed hungry, and never go to bed on an over-full stomach. Too little food and that gnawing pang in the pit of your stomach will certainly make sure that you have a restless night of fitful sleep. Too much and you will suffer indigestion, heartburn, flatulence and again a disturbed night.

If you suffer from an hiatus hernia, you need to take special care with your evening eating habits. This condition, in which the opening in the diaphragm through which the oesophagus (food tube) passes becomes too loose and allows the acid contents of the stomach to leak upwards into the oesophagus, causes most disruption at night-time. As soon as you lie down, the presence of stomach acids in the wrong place causes severe heartburn and considerable pain.

There are practical steps which minimise this disruptive discomfort. Raise the head end of your bed by about 4 in

(10 cm), using proper bed blocks or a brick under each leg. Do not drink any liquids at all less than three hours before bedtime. Do not eat large meals in the evening. And avoid pickles, vinegar, acidic foods and anything fried.

There is some evidence that malted milk drinks like Horlicks and Ovaltine really do help to encourage better sleep. The beneficial effects are more apparent in older people, and the main benefits seem to be during the later stages of sleep rather than in getting to sleep in the first place. If you find that you drop off easily, but wake in the small hours, it's certainly worth trying either of these drinks about half an hour before bedtime.

Honey has long been a favourite folk remedy for insomnia. Take it mixed with a little warm milk, in a cup of chamomile tea or in hot water with lemon. And don't forget all the other soothing herbal remedies (see page 89).

There is no denying that we are what we eat and you cannot expect a good night's sleep if you are constantly consuming large quantities of coffee, tea, chocolate or cola drinks, which all supply your brain with a constant stream of irritating caffeine. You won't sleep if you're hungry. You're unlikely to sleep after a take-away snack of pie, chips and three pickled onions. As far as food is concerned, the watch-words should be: not too little, not too much, but just right. What is just right for you, you will find by trial and error.

8

SNORING – THE MAJOR CAUSE OF OTHER PEOPLE'S INSOMNIA AND A HEALTH HAZARD TO THE SNORER

'There ain't no way to find out why a snorer can't hear himself snore.'

Mark Twain

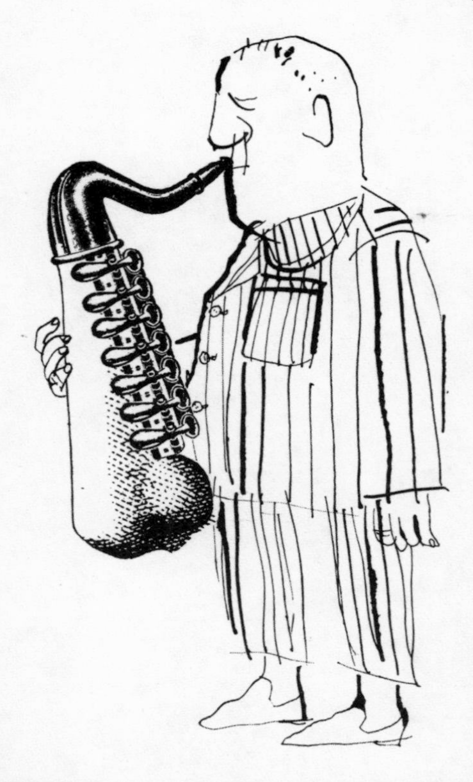

Nobody quite knows why it is predominantly men that snore, but the fact is that 20% of men and only 5% of women under the age of 35 snore. By the time we get to 60, 60% of men and 40% of women are regular snorers. Maybe there is a grain of truth in the old legend that our caveman ancestors learned to snore as a way of frightening off marauding wild animals, thus protecting their womenfolk even while they slept. It seems a shame that in our modern society the effect is to keep away the women, for as Anthony Burgess wrote in *Inside Mr Enderby*, 'Laugh and the world laughs with you; snore and you sleep alone.' Apart from the obvious physical problems of damage to the nose and deformities which may cause snoring, the prime suspects in this detective story are being overweight or drinking alcohol, or, worst of all, a combination of both. Statistically the overweight are three times more likely to snore than their thin counterparts.

It's a strange fact that a condition which causes so much stress to some people should be the cause of so much hilarity to everybody else. No matter how disturbed your life is by sharing it with a snorer, everybody else seems to treat the problem as a joke. It's always the partner or the neighbour or the person in the next door hotel room that complains, and never the snorer. He is convinced that all the tales of his window-shattering emissions are exaggerated figments of other people's imagination. After all, if the noise was really that bad how could he possibly have slept through it, being such a light sleeper that even the cat padding down the hallway is enough to wake him up? He lives in a world of self-delusion. Some of the record-breaking snorers have produced noises which exceed legal limits. The current *Guinness Book of Records* reveals that Mark Hubbard from Richmond, Canada, is the world's best snorer. At peak levels his nocturnal emissions, measured at the Department of Medicine in Vancouver, reached 90 decibels. Mark queried whether he was legally entitled to sleep in the city of Vancouver as the city traffic law limit for noise is a mere 80 decibels.

The men don't have it all their own way. Florence Phillips, an 87-year-old widow from Leeds, was recently mentioned in *The Times,* when local magistrates came to the conclusion that the terrible racket of her snoring was in contravention of the Control of Pollution Act.

But, when all's said and done, there is a serious side to snoring. It really is highly disruptive to the sleep of both the snorer and the innocent party. The latter for obvious reasons; when earplugs, personal stereos and elbows in the ribs fail, it often means a shift to another bedroom and, to all intents and purposes, an end to physical relationships. This in itself does little for the sleeping habits of either partner, although escape from the sound of a Harley Davidson two inches from your ear must be worth almost any price.

The adverse effects on the snorer are less obvious, though often far more serious. An increasingly recognised complaint is that of sleep apnoea, a condition which gets its name from the Greek word for breathlessness. Originally this condition was thought to be rare and associated with serious respiratory or central nervous diseases. Observations in sleep laboratories have now confirmed that it is common in habitual snorers, and far more so in obese habitual snorers. The subject falls asleep normally, usually to the accompaniment of a few loud snorts, and then settles to the normal regular pattern of snoring. The soft tissues at the back of the throat tend to fold inwards and, especially in overweight people who are more likely to suffer from nasal obstructions and smaller airways, the flow of inspiration is cut off. Breathing stops for anything from 30 seconds to a minute. The brain then panics, as it needs a continual supply of oxygen in order to survive. It sends messages to rouse you from your stupor; to stimulate the diaphragm and the other breathing muscles, you take a couple of violent snorting breaths and settle back to your regular rhythm. This can be repeated dozens of times throughout the night, and each episode almost wakes you up. The resulting disturbance of sleep produces early morning headaches and feelings of tiredness the following day. Heavy snorers with this problem may well find themselves nodding off at work, sometimes in the most embarrassing situations, and even more worryingly they are at serious risk of falling asleep at the wheel while driving – a risk that is even greater when faced with the monotony of motorways.

For any watcher this can be a frightening condition, as it may seem that the snorer is not going to breathe again. Rarely he may not, since this pattern of breathing puts extreme stress on the heart and circulatory system and can lead to irregular heart beat, which in the presence of any existing heart disease may be fatal. Anyone who suffers from apnoea should see their doctor in order to exclude any serious underlying illness. In the absence of any such disease, the serious snorer should see an ENT specialist, as there are simple surgical procedures which may be applicable. This is even more important where sleep apnoea is a regular problem. Snoring children may also suffer the same problem and this is sometimes related to enlarged tonsils or adenoids. Happily the routine removal of these important organs is no longer fashionable, but apnoea can affect a child's performance at school and lack of sleep on a long-term basis is also likely to produce personality changes. In this situation surgery can produce dramatic improvements.

Alcohol certainly compounds the problem and poses a serious threat to the snorer with apnoea. Likewise all the benzodiazepine tranquillisers will make the condition worse and must be avoided.

Kill or Cure

Snoring can be fatal, not just as a result of apnoea, but because of the intense rage which it generates in others. Threats of physical violence are far from uncommon, and in the USA murder has been committed. The great western gunslinger, John Wesley Hardin, was reputedly so infuriated by the snores coming from the next door hotel room that he pulled his gun and shot the culprit through the wall. There was even a report from Dallas in the 1980s that the police had arrested a woman who used a pistol, which she had hidden in the bed, to shoot a male companion because his snoring was so loud.

There are a number of things you must do if you are a snorer, which will improve matters. There are also lots of ideas that are worth trying. They may not help but they can't hurt, and just by making an effort you'll show your partner that you understand her plight and are prepared to try.

Being fat is an almost certain cause of snoring – there are lots of thin people who snore but very few obese ones who don't. The first step is to lose some weight, and you can do this with the diet plan on page 36. Next, cut down on the alcohol, or better still don't take any at all in the evening. Avoid tranquillisers and, above all, absolutely avoid tranquillisers and alcohol together. Start taking some regular exercise. This will improve your breathing as well as your overall fitness and help with the weight loss. Give up smoking. This may seem obvious and boring, but smoking affects your breathing and is likely to cause bronchitis or other serious chronic respiratory diseases. This makes it more likely that you will suffer from apnoea, and the sort of airways obstruction which makes your snoring worse.

Snoring is nearly always worse when you sleep on your back, and a simple solution is to clip two or three of the spring-type clothes pegs to the centre of the back of your pyjama jacket. As an alternative, you could sew a tennis ball into the back of the jacket. Both of these are uncomfortable to lie on, so when, having gone to sleep on your side, you, as is inevitable, turn over in your sleep and end up on your back, the discomfort will soon make you turn back again without waking up.

For those who only wear Armani cologne in bed, there are some electronic gadgets which can do the trick. These are sensitive to the noise and vibration of snoring. They are fixed to the wrist like a watch and when triggered stimulate the skin with an electronic buzz. This is enough to disturb your sleep so that you move and stop snoring. The machine then switches off till you snore again.

Lack of humidity dries out the mucous membranes of the nose and throat and will aggravate snoring. If you have a radiator in your bedroom hang a humidifier over it – a wet towel will do, but you can buy small electric humidifiers which consume very little electricity and make no noise.

Some snoring can be due to allergies. Pollen and other airborne irritants, or some foods, can cause swelling of the mucous membranes, overproduction of mucus, and consequent difficulties with breathing. Make sure that the bedroom is thoroughly cleaned with a vacuum cleaner each day. Pay particular attention to ledges, window sills, the top of the wardrobe, the bed-head, and the bed itself. Wipe all surfaces where dust can settle with a damp cloth as near to bedtime as possible. Avoid long pile carpets, elaborately pleated curtains and bedspreads, and keep bedrooms as cool as possible, turning off radiators in the winter. Do not let any animals into the bedroom and least of all on to the bed. If your snorer suffers from allergies it's worth putting an ioniser and an air filter into the bedroom. There are small machines available which do both these jobs at once, and can produce noticeable improvements in the air quality, and, consequently, in the snoring.

Food allergies are another common trigger. For some people milk can be a real problem, causing overproduction of mucus and congestion of the nose and sinuses. This makes snoring worse. Other culprits include many of the artificial food additives, colourings and flavourings, particularly monosodium glutamate and the yellow, red and green colours.

Finally, don't forget the value of some of the aromatic herbs and essential oils (see page 94). These can help to dilate the passages in the airways and improve breathing. You can sprinkle a little on the pillow, rub some on the chest, spray it in the air, or even use a small burner to vaporise the oils. The best of all the commercially available products is a wonderful spray called Climarome. This is made by the famous French aromatherapist, Dr Jean Valnet, and not only smells wonderful, but is extremely effective. Make sure that you eat plenty of garlic as this is another of nature's powerful decongestants. If you really can't bear the taste, take six Kwai Garlic tablets each day. These are made from the whole dried garlic and they are specially coated so that you don't taste them or smell of them.

One consolation for the snorer's partner is that in time, and with perseverance, it is possible to get used to the most extraordinary noises without them disrupting your sleep. In fact, the reverse is true. People living on the end of the runway at Heathrow, or with a railway at the bottom of the garden, are constantly amazed by visitors who exclaim the next morning, 'How do you sleep with all that noise?' The normal response is 'What noise?' and more often than not sleep is disrupted when the regular noises stop – when there is fog at the airport or a strike on the railways.

You may find it hard to believe if you have just acquired a snoring partner, but in my researches I have found people who can't sleep when their snorer is away from home – they miss the comforting knowledge that their other half is close by them.

9

SEX AND RELAXATION – THE ULTIMATE SOLUTION TO ALL SLEEP PROBLEMS, ONE OR THE OTHER BUT BEST OF ALL BOTH

'*Sleep* – Of all the soft, delicious functions of nature this is the chiefest; what a happiness it is to man, when the anxieties and passions of the day are over.'

Lawrence Sterne

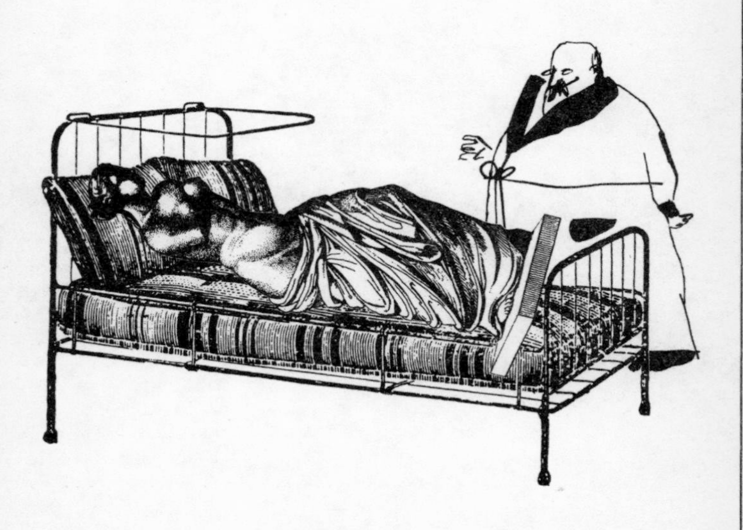

You can't open a newspaper, read a magazine or turn on the radio today without hearing something about stress. And most of it is pretty bad. Not all stress, however, is bad. Our responses to stress are what have enabled us to survive as a species. Where we get into trouble is when we can't respond in the proper way to stress. The fright, fight and flight syndrome I've already mentioned is the key to the entire problem. When man is exposed to some sort of unpleasant stimulus, his body reacts by producing vast quantities of a chemical called adrenalin, and this prepares us either to run away or to fight back. In modern society we are constantly subjected to a bombardment of stimuli and nearly always are unable to act in the appropriate way. If you have a disagreement with your boss at work, you can't run away, you can't fight back. If you work in a shop and you are dealing with a difficult customer, you have to grit your teeth and grin and bear it.

This is the sort of stress which creates problems, because all this unused adrenalin builds up in the system, causes muscle tension, makes the blood pressure go up and creates all the possible problems of these two effects. The excessive adrenalin interferes with normal patterns of sleep and when mixed with the emotional turmoil that unresolved problems leave behind, insomnia becomes almost inevitable. Stress can also be responsible for many physical symptoms, aches and pains, high blood pressure, which can result in heart disease, a stroke and all sorts of debilitating problems; migraine, skin diseases, asthma, even some other allergies are directly linked to excessive stress.

It is not possible or even desirable to avoid stress. Stress permeates the society in which we live, so unless you're prepared to become a hermit and cut yourself off totally from civilisation, you'd better learn how to cope with stress and how to use it to your advantage. Don't forget that it is stress which puts the edge on performance, heightens the sense of awareness, quickens the reflexes and sharpens the wits.

The great trick is to learn how to master the way in which stress affects your body and to minimise the physical side effects it causes; to understand the mechanisms which transfer undesirable messages from your brain to your body. The power of the mind to cause psychosomatic illness is huge and should never be underestimated; primitive man has understood and used this power for thousands of years. The literature is peppered with accounts of witch doctors' curses leading to the unpreventable death of their victims. The investigation of modern drugs is always done with the use of placebo studies and the placebo effect can be dramatic. One group of patients is given the real drug, another a totally inert medicine which looks, smells and tastes just the same. In most trials results show that the fake pill often works almost as well as the genuine one, at least for the first two or three months.

There are lots of ways in which you can put your mind and body to work and start the process of separating emotional stress and physical discomfort. The first step is to learn how to relax.

One of the commonest side effects of stress is muscle tension. The body very quickly adapts to new patterns of muscle tone and what for a small child would be unbearably uncomfortable, becomes the the norm for the adult subjected to repetitive stresses. You get used to your own body's stresses and in fact there are many people who get addicted to stress. The typical example of the weekend migraine used to be the preserve of busy executive businessmen, but with more and more women taking on high-powered and demanding jobs, it's just as common with businesswomen too. You struggle through the week coping with problems, with excesses, with difficulties. The minute you get home on Friday evening and unwind, the migraine starts. A stress reaction.

With practice it's possible to learn how to teach your body to reawaken its awareness of relaxation and to be more aware of the discomforts of muscular stress and strain. The easiest way to achieve this is by recreating muscle fatigue. The important thing is to give yourself time – allow yourself half an hour at the end of the day. Make yourself comfortable. These exercises are best done lying flat on the floor, on a nice thick rug or a thin foam mattress, the sort of thing you have on a sun lounger or for camping. Wrap yourself in a light, thin but warm blanket, take the telephone off the hook, lock the door, draw the blinds and shut yourself away from the demands of the outside world. And this includes husbands, wives, parents, children, neighbours – shut them all out and give yourself half an hour to relearn the natural way of coping with stress.

Read through the exercises a couple of times just to get the feel of the routine. Then put on a favourite piece of soothing music, make sure it lasts at least half an hour (if not compile your own tape) and ideally get someone else to read the instructions to you slowly and very quietly. If this is not possible, record them on tape yourself and play them back through a personal stereo, but don't forget to speak the instructions slowly and to leave pauses in which to do the exercises.

What we're going to do is to take your body through a series of muscle contractions and relaxations, exerting those muscles in such a way that at the end of the series of exercises the muscles will be suffering fatigue. The result of this fatigue is complete and total relaxation. So, lie flat on the floor, making sure that you're comfortable and warm, with a small pillow under your head, and loose clothing. Let's begin.

I want you to close your eyes, and I want you to start by stretching your left leg as hard as you can away from your body. Push it down, keeping it in contact with the floor, pointing your toes and contracting all the muscles of the calf and thigh and pointing your toes down as hard as you can. Really push, don't let go yet, keep holding on to those muscles. And relax. Now let's do the same thing with the right leg. Push that leg straight down along the floor away from your trunk, point the toes down, contract the calf muscles and really squeeze the muscles of your thigh. Push hard, don't let go yet, keep pushing. Keep pushing with that leg, and relax. Now let's push both legs together, push down as hard as you can. Push those legs away from your trunk, point the toes down, squeeze the calf muscles, squeeze the thigh muscles, feel your bottom muscles squeezing as hard as you can. Keep pushing, keep pushing, your muscles are probably starting to tremble a little bit now – that's good. Don't let go yet, don't stop breathing. And relax.

Now let's do the same thing with the left arm. I want you to push your left arm as hard as you can down along the side of your body. Push the hand towards the feet, spread your fingers as wide as you can. Press down with the shoulder muscles, contract the arm muscles, contract the shoulder muscles. Push as hard as you can. Don't let go yet – keep pushing, keep pushing. And relax. Now let's do the same thing with the right arm. Push the arm as hard as you can along your side towards your right foot. Spread the fingers as wide as possible, feel the muscles of the forearm contracting. Press with the shoulder, keep pressing, keep breathing. You don't have to stop breathing. Keep pressing with that arm. And relax. Now let's press both arms. Stretch them down from the shoulders, stretch hard, spread the fingers as wide as you can. Feel those forearm muscles contracting, feel your biceps and your triceps, keep pressing, spread the fingers, spread the fingers. Are your muscles trembling? You're doing it right. Keep pressing, and relax.

Now, we're going to press everything together. I want you to stretch your legs and arms as hard as you can, and push. Stretch the legs down, push the arms down, with your hands reaching towards your feet. Point the toes down, contract the calf muscles, squeeze the bottom muscles, push with the shoulders, spread the fingers as wide as possible. Hold it all like that, but do keep breathing. Push a little harder, wait for those muscles to start trembling. Keep pushing, don't give up yet, just a little bit harder. And relax. Take a very deep breath in. Breathe in . . . fill your lungs, expand your chest as far as you can, and push the breath out. And breathe in again, as far as you can, a little bit more, stretch your ribcage, hold your breath, and push it out. One more deep, deep breath. Breathe in . . . hold your breath . . . and breathe out. Now we'll do it all again.

Let's start with the left leg. Stretch your left leg down from your trunk, point the toe, squeeze the calf muscle, contract the thigh muscles, and push. Keep holding it, push as hard as you can. Keep pushing, keep pushing. And relax the leg. Now the right leg. Push, push, push, point the toe, squeeze the calf muscles, squeeze the thigh muscles. Feel that leg really begin to tremble now. Keep pushing, keep pushing, hold it still, don't stop breathing. And relax the leg. Now let's do both legs together. And push as hard as you can. Point the toes down, squeeze the calf muscles, feel your buttock muscles squeezing as hard as they possibly can. Push with the thigh muscles, keep pushing with those legs, keep breathing and push, and push, and make those legs tremble with the effort of using the muscles. Keep pushing, and relax.

Now the left arm, push down from the shoulder, stretch the fingers as wide as you can, push the hand towards the left foot. Feel those shoulder muscles, feel the muscles in your forearm, hold them steady, hold it, don't let go yet. Keep pushing, keep pushing, and relax. And now, the right arm. Push down, stretch the fingers, push from the shoulder, feel those forearm muscles, feel the arm beginning to tremble. Keep breathing, keep breathing, don't let go of that arm yet. Keep pushing, and relax. Now both arms again, push down, stretch the fingers as far as possible, feel the shoulders pushing down, feel the forearm muscles, push with the biceps, push with the triceps. Hold both arms, keep pushing, keep pushing, if those arms aren't trembling you aren't pushing hard enough. Keep pushing and keep breathing. Hold it, hold it steady. And relax again.

Now, let's have both arms and both legs together, and a big, big push with everything. Push with the arms, push with the shoulders, spread those fingers a little wider. Point those toes down as far as you can. Feel the buttock muscles contracting, squeeze the calves, push with the thigh muscles, spread the fingers. Hold everything just like that and push just as hard as you can. Don't stop breathing, keep pushing, keep pushing, keep pushing hard – everything should be trembling nicely. Keep pushing, and relax again.

Take a deep, deep breath in, breathe in . . ., fill those lungs up, expand your chest, and push the breath out. And another deep breath in . . ., right in, as far as you can, and just a little bit further, push that oxygen into your lungs, and breathe right out . . . And one more really deep, deep breath, breathe in . . . a little bit more, a little bit more, hold your breath, and very slowly let the breath out as gently as you can . . . right out . . . right out. And just rest where you are for a moment.

Doesn't that feel good? All the tensions just wash away. The stresses of the day, breathed out with your last slow breath. As with any form of exercise, if you are really going to benefit from these simple relaxation techniques, you have to practise.

Now, I want you to do the same sequence of exercises another three times. Don't forget, it's left leg, right leg, both legs together, left arm, right arm, both arms together, and then arms and legs at the same time. Don't forget to breathe while you're pushing, and don't forget to take three really deep breaths in and out between each group of exercises. The more you practise, the easier it becomes. When you've done five sequences of this exercise you will feel beautifully and peacefully relaxed. In time you will be able to achieve the same degree of relaxation with just one sequence of exercises, or maybe with just the very thought of relaxation.

What you will achieve if you persevere is the establishing of a new reflex pattern. Just thinking the word 'relax' will trigger the conditioned response that you have built up by repetition, and you will be able to invoke that response sitting in a traffic jam, in the dentist's chair, in fact in any stressful situation. It won't make the stress go away, but it will prevent the build-up of tension which gives you sleepless nights.

We all have a great need to relax and it's not enough just to have a couple of weeks' holiday in the sunshine once a year. (In fact, going on holiday is one of the more stressful activities, particularly since it is often the longest period of time which families spend together during the whole twelve months.) It is essential to learn to relax consciously for short periods every day, and this does not mean going to sleep in the armchair in front of the TV. Being relaxed is a conscious state in which the muscles are free of tension and the brain free of disturbing thoughts.

For some people activity is the key to this state, they can achieve it by playing a sport, or digging the garden; others prefer to relax passively by reading, listening to music or watching the TV. The first two are fine but the images on the small screen can either lull you off to sleep in a thoroughly uncomfortable position which is likely to give you a pain in the back or neck, or the programme may be overstimulating and agitating, which defeats the object of the exercise.

When you achieve a state of relaxation your body goes through a number of specific changes. You may enjoy a sense of heightened awareness, sensations of warmth and heaviness will spread through your muscles. Your heartbeat slows down, the level of both sugar and fat in your bloodstream falls, and your whole system seems to drop into a lower gear. Since the effects of stress are exactly the reverse, raised blood pressure, blood sugar, blood fats and heartbeat, it's obvious that the benefits of relaxation are far-reaching in both physical and emotional terms.

There are a number of specific techniques as well as the exercises above which can be used successfully to deal with stress problems which are causing insomnia. We've already discussed the value of massage (see page 93) and the importance of exercise (see page 32). Here we shall consider some of the psychological and contemplative techniques which are easy to learn and extremely effective. Like all other skills, they need practice if you are going to succeed.

Hypnosis can be remarkably effective in overcoming the bane of insomnia. Like all therapies it does not work for every subject in every situation, but in the proper hands it's safe, comparatively simple and certainly worth trying.

Most people seem to believe that the conscious mind is the most important. It appears to be in charge of everything we think and do, whilst the unconscious looks after all the functions that we are not aware of. In fact the reverse is true and the subconscious mind never stops working to control all the functions of both mind and body. The conscious switches off when we sleep, the unconscious doesn't. The subconscious is a vast databank which is our memory, storing away every single detail of every day.

During hypnosis the therapist is able to communicate directly with the subconscious mind while the subject is in a resting state of limbo. Hypnosis does not put you to sleep, it merely reduces awareness of your surroundings and, so to speak, turns down the volume control of the conscious mind. In this state the hypnotist can give suggestions directly into the subconscious mind which it will accept without question.

The value of hypnosis lies in its ability to change behaviour patterns and control physiological functions. Its value in the treatment of insomnia lies in its ability to help with physical discomforts, like pain, and with emotional difficulties, like stress and anxiety. This helps to remove the obstacles to sleep and restore normal patterns.

Contrary to popular belief, there are no dark rooms or

swinging pocket watches, and in fact hypnosis is a very pleasant therapy. There is an added bonus in that you will almost certainly learn more about coping with life and learning to relax than is needed just for the relief of your sleeping problems. The benefits of this treatment will have wide-reaching applications beyond your insomnia.

Autogenic training is a system of mental exercises developed by the German specialist Dr Schultz in the 1930s. It consists of a system of mental exercises which are done to help overcome both mental and physical stress. The object of this exercise is to override the body's normal stress responses – the fright, fight or flight reflex which produces adrenalin. It replaces this response by switching into the body's rest, relaxation and recreation mode. It's called autogenic because its name derives from the word autogenous which means self-generating. The technique comes from within the body itself and is one which can easily be learnt from a qualified practitioner.

You'll be taught to experience a variety of sensations like warmth and heaviness of the limbs. You'll learn to regulate the heartbeat and respiration. You will be able to produce feelings of coolness of the forehead and warmth in the stomach. All this is achieved by repeating instructions over and over again, and once you have learned the technique it can bring relief from stress and anxiety. It will help you to cope with current problems and to eradicate physical tensions which have developed over long periods of time.

Biofeedback is a training system which uses electronic technology to help you learn how to control many of your body responses. The instruments are able to measure skin temperature, muscle tone, or even the amount of acid being produced in your stomach.

The easiest measurement is that of the amount of sweat which your skin is producing. Anxiety, as we all know, increases sweating, and by attaching electrical contacts to the skin and connecting them to a machine which generates variable pitch noises or different coloured lights, it becomes possible for the subject to see or hear the responses caused by the amount of stress and anxiety present. With sufficient practice it is possible to learn how to control all your stress responses so that eventually you no longer need the machinery.

Biofeedback is increasingly used in mainstream medicine and has particular value in the relief of high blood pressure, migraine, heart conditions and, of course, insomnia.

Meditation has always formed one of the major foundation stones of Indian religions and Tibetan Buddhism. The object of meditation is the balance and harmony between reality and idealism and though there are many different forms of meditation, they all share to some extent or other three basic concepts:-

A clear appreciation of the perfect order of things which is developed through greater awareness.

The development of a state of mind which is receptive to that perfect order.

Active participation in putting the theory of that order into practice.

Successful meditation depends on the ability to develop the special state of awareness, a situation of restful alertness during which it's possible to empty the mind. This is usually achieved by focusing your concentration on an object, a flower, a mark on the wall, a distant tree, anything in fact which you find suitable, and at the same time repeating over and over again a particular phrase, word or sound, which is known as a mantra. Once mastered, this skill will make it infinitely easier to cope with stress, anxiety and tension and, practised on a regular basis, especially at night-time, it is yet another weapon in the fight against sleep deprivation.

There are lots of good books on meditation but it is always easier to learn any of these techniques from a competent teacher. If you would like to have a go at learning for yourself, the following exercise is a compilation of a variety of meditative practices which has been developed by Dr Herbert Benson at Harvard Medical School. It's a simple distillation of 1,000 years of eastern wisdom, and you may find it of great value in overcoming your problem.

Sit, lie or recline in a comfortable position, making sure there are no external distractions such as radio or television.

Shut your eyes.

Relax all your muscles as in the basic relaxation exercise described earlier.

Breathe deeply through your nose and try to clear your mind of all thought. Repeat the mantra word, 'one', either aloud or in your head. Breathe deeply and evenly and continue for 10–20 minutes, ignoring distracting thoughts and repeating the mantra.

At the end, remain still, with your eyes shut for one or two minutes, then in the same position with your eyes open.

Some forms of meditation can cause sudden outbursts of emotion, such as tears or laughter. This is said to be a sign that the meditation is working.

Yoga is generally used as a generic name which encompasses a variety of relaxing exercises combined with meditation and a variety of poses. Although it is a part of some eastern religions, the techniques in themselves, even when separated from their religious connotations, provide an excellent way of coping with life's slings and arrows. Half an hour of yoga each day can work more effectively, more safely and more permanently than a bottle full of sleeping pills.

The practical benefits of yoga also include improved mobility and flexibility, it promotes inner harmony and reduces both stress and tension leading to sound sleep and a deep sense of relaxation.

Age is no bar to taking up yoga, and it makes no difference whether you are eight or 80, fit or not. I advise many of my older patients to take up yoga as it is a gentle form of exercise suitable even for those suffering from rheumatism and arthritis. A good teacher will make sure that you only perform movements which are within your physical capabilities, and these movements are highly beneficial to anyone with joint problems. This is another therapy which is best learnt from an expert teacher and though frustrating to begin with, you will be surprised at how quickly your ability to adopt the yoga poses develops.

There are many people for whom stress-related insomnia cannot be solved just through taking physical exercise or enjoying their hobbies. For them it is common for the additional benefit of physical relaxation to be the missing piece in the jigsaw.

I urge you to experiment with all these forms of relaxation therapy until you find the one that suits you best. Even if your insomnia is temporary and you know its cause, the importance of learning how to relax is far wider than just conquering your sleep disorder. None of us can avoid episodes of stress in our lives and the ability to overcome that stress and to dissipate its harmful side effects will stand you in good stead throughout life.

Sex can be both a cause and cure of sleeplessness. The frustrations of the denied or unfulfilled partner, the sadness of the lonely single person, the pinings of the adolescent, the yearnings of the romantic – all these conspire to rob you of your slumbers. The woman subjected to the uncaring demands of a selfish partner; the couple who never talk about sex, only ever do it on Saturday night with the lights out in bed, and neither of whom derives either sexual or emotional satisfaction from the act; the male whose partner regards intercourse as an unpleasant favour to be bestowed as and when she feels he's earned the right, are all unlikely to fall asleep feeling warm and contented.

Sex can be a minefield, but properly handled it can also be a boon. Being single and alone is no bar. Masturbation does not make you blind or sap your energy, and is a perfectly normal and acceptable form of human behaviour to be enjoyed without shame or guilt. It's particularly important for women who have passed the menopause and find themselves, as is so often the case, the sole survivor of a marriage. Regular sex and orgasms help to stimulate the flow of hormones which play a large part in the body's mechanism for manufacturing bone cells. For this reason alone it is a good thing for older women to enjoy regular sexual activity and satisfaction, as well as for the benefits it brings in the form of better sleep. If you are in this predicament why not buy a vibrator: they work.

Many women complain to me that their lovemaking is unsatisfactory. As punk musician Johnny Rotten said, 'Love is two minutes 52 seconds of squishing noises'. Immediately 'he' has had his orgasm he rolls over and goes to sleep and never questions whether 'I' have had one too, or have even enjoyed the whole experience. No one would suggest that this is love-making, it is only selfish gratification. In a living and caring relationship intercourse is more than just a physical act. It is a time of close communication, of sharing and caring for your partner. It's at this time that the warmth and tenderness can engulf and override all the reasons for not sleeping.

The release of hormones generated by the physical act of making love, together with the muscular fatigue which follows, should induce a wonderful glow of well-being, peace and comfort which will lead naturally into sound sleep.

One of the great pioneers of modern childbirth, the French obstetrician Frederick Leboyer said, 'Making love is the sovereign remedy for anguish.' Remember that the next time someone tries to tell you that sex keeps you awake.

If you want to achieve the ultimate in good sleep, then try a combination of the relaxation techniques and sex. Start with some massage, as this will produce feelings of closeness and intimacy. Then if, and only if, it's obviously what you both want, let things take their natural course. You will be amazed by the difference which, starting from a more relaxed base, you will notice in the myriad of emotional and physical sensations experienced during the course of your love-making. You will sleep and wake the next morning refreshed and with the sense of muscular ease which has eluded you for so long.

There's no point in expecting these intimate adventures to be a roaring success if you've got to the end of a fraught and difficult day, collapse into bed and indulge in a bit of quick nookie of the 'wham bam thank you ma'am' type. Take a little time to use one of the other forms of relaxation and for the best results do it together. This does not mean that yoga, meditation, relaxation exercises or any of the others should become a necessary prelude to sex, nor that sex should become the inevitable sequel to the relaxation. Use both activities in their own right, and when appropriate you'll find that combining the two provides ample proof that the value of the whole is equal to far more than the sum of the individual parts.

10

SLEEPLESS CHILDREN

'Slepe is the nourishment and food of a sucking child'

Thomas Phaer

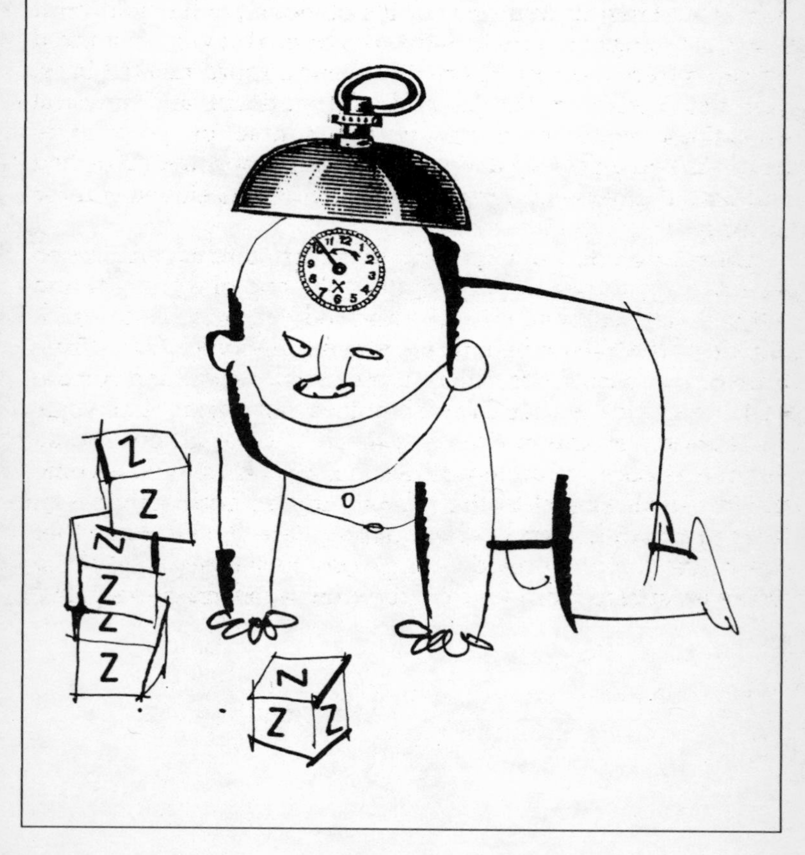

The sleep requirement of babies, infants and small children are not only different from each other and fall into different patterns, but they are all different from normal adult needs. One thing, however, is certain, and that is that interrupted nights have far more effect on the parents than they do on the offspring.

It's all too easy for mothers in particular to believe that the sleepless baby or toddler is in some way a reflection on her maternal qualities. She's likely to feel guilty that her child is difficult to get to sleep, or impossible to keep asleep during the night. This in turn disturbs the father who is likely to complain that he 'has to get up to go to work in the morning', adding further to the feelings of guilt. In spite of all the media suggestions to the contrary, in my experience the 'modern' man is more an inhabitant of the ad agency's creative department than of real life. The reality seems to be that 'macho man' is still alive and well and living in Surbiton, Milton Keynes, Swansea, Newcastle, Lands End, John O'Groats, and everywhere between.

Bringing up children is a joint effort. Fathers who don't take an active part in the humdrum business of nappy changing, bottle-warming and night duty miss out on a great deal of the joys of parenthood as well as not relieving mothers of some of the trials and tribulations. In our society where so many young mothers also go to work as well as looking after home and children, it becomes even more important that the chores as well as the pleasures of parenthood should be more equally divided.

The new-born do not come from identical moulds like rows of jelly babies. Every one is an individual with its own temperament, likes, dislikes and distinctive behaviour patterns. It's unrealistic to expect that every child will follow the same patterns of sleep; after all adults don't, so there is no reason to think there is anything wrong with your baby just because it doesn't seem to sleep as your mother-in-law says it should. The majority of sleep disorders in babies and children can be explained and overcome and this is an essential need. Three or four years of broken nights, anxiety and frustration will wreak havoc in the best of relationships and may be a common cause of violence directed at the luckless infant. I've heard the most even-tempered, responsible and loving mothers talking about their fear of 'doing something terrible to the baby' when they are in a state of mental and physical exhaustion following night after night of sleeplessness. These poor women get to the end of their tether, they suffer depression, anxiety and even breakdown, all of which can be at worst considerably reduced, and at best eliminated, by a better understanding of the problem and a more holistic approach to its solutions.

Twenty years ago, when my son Alexander was just three months old, we had a family visit to New York. Being very short of time and wanting to see as much as possible I hired a car and driver for the day and one of our stops was at the Metropolitan Museum. Unfortunately they wouldn't allow us to take the baby buggy into the building and the thought of carrying a hefty baby for a couple of hours almost made us change our minds. Our driver, an archetypal New York Irish cabbie, said he was quite happy to wait outside with the baby in his carry-cot. Imagine our horror when, two hours later, we came out of the museum to find no sign of taxi, driver or son. Every bad story about New York flashed before our eyes like the drowning man's dream. Just as we were debating whether to find a policeman, the taxi came cruising round the corner and our smiling driver leapt out to explain that Alexander had started screaming. As a father of eight and grandfather of 13, he knew just what to do – 'I drove him round the block with some nice music on the radio and he was asleep in ten minutes.'

This lesson stood us in good stead. Alexander was a wonderful sleeper and gave us very few broken nights. His younger sister, Tanya, was a different story. She kept us awake on and off for three years, and many's the night that she has been driven around in the back of a car, sometimes for five minutes, sometimes for half an hour, before finally dropping off to sleep. Her mother and I blessed our New York taxi driver a thousand times.

In hindsight it's easy to realise that, like many parents, our attempts to solve the problem had been pathetic and ill-informed. I'm sure that by the end our youngest had learned to enjoy her nocturnal car journeys and found that all she had to do to get one was to lie in bed and scream. On the other hand, some expert advice had been to let her scream. We tried it once. She screamed for two hours, and for days we lived in dread of the police or social workers turning up on the doorstep in response to some nosey neighbour's reporting of a local case of baby battering.

Every parent willingly endures the occasional sleepless night, sitting up with a sick child, soothing away a nightmare, coping with over-excitement or anxiety. These intermittent interruptions to our own sleep don't pose a problem as they rarely extend beyond one or two bad nights at a time. Continuous sleep-deprivation presents a totally awesome problem, not for the child, who will certainly make up for it by dozing during the day, but for the parent who has to continue functioning at home or at work. All the current research demonstrates the long-term effects of sleep-deprivation. Even when the desperate parent tries going to bed at nine at night and possibly achieves nine hours sleeping time, the value of that sleep when it is constantly interrupted is negligible even when compared to five or six hours of continuous sleep. Although the latter may be too little for many people, the effects which this has are minimal, apart from feelings of fatigue. Constantly disturbed sleep leads to loss of concentration, irritability, feelings of anger and frustration and depression, all well known to the parents of non-sleeping children.

Sleep disorders and their causes vary with the age of the child, as do the solutions. But as a parent you must be aware that the attempts of many health-care professionals, to say nothing of in-laws, friends and neighbours, to lay the blame at your doorstep are almost always totally misguided. Somehow the impression given to the poor, long-suffering mother is that just because 'they' never produced sleepless children, 'you' must be doing something wrong. Do not let them convince you – very few babies perform just like it says they should in the book.

What is true is that the way in which problems are dealt with can affect the length of time it takes to resolve them, and hopefully the guidance that follows will get you on the best possible course to solving the difficulties in the shortest possible time. If it doesn't work for you and your child, don't blame yourself, but keep searching for other ideas to try. Be careful not to fall into the 'I've tried everything' syndrome, which usually means you've tried everything for a day or two, and not tried anything for long enough to see if it works. If your family has suffered broken nights for a year already, you can't expect a magic wand to put everything back to normal in 24 hours. Persevere and be prepared to wait for a gradual solution.

The New Baby

During their first weeks of life babies spend most of their time sleeping, roughly the same amount day and night, and they can usually be expected to wake every three or four hours. With luck many will sleep through most of the night by the time they reach six or seven weeks. There is not very much difference in the total sleeping time between new babies and older ones. What does change is the pattern of their sleep. A new baby will actually be asleep for roughly 16 hours in each 24; by four months the total sleep time has only fallen to around 14 hours, but by then you would expect to be seeing eight-hour stretches of continuous sleep. By the time a child reaches one year most of them will have settled into a routine of two or possibly three periods of sleep during any one day, and by the age of three many children will only want to sleep at night time. Just to show how contrary children are, there are some who, even at the age of five or six, will still want a nap in the afternoon.

If your child does not fit exactly with these figures, don't panic, remember they are only averages and not normals. None of them is a holy writ any deviation from which is an indication that you are a bad parent, that your child is slow, bright, dull, intelligent, or psychologically deprived.

As we've already seen in Chapter 1, as well as fitting into the circadian rhythm of the 24-hour day, adults sleep in the ultradian rhythm of 100-minute cycles. In babies this cycle is only of 50 minutes' duration. Consequently, babies have more periods of light sleep during any given night than do adults. Given this fact it's not surprising that babies wake more often. A well-fed, warm and dry baby may go through anything from one to four of these cycles without making demands on its parents, so it could sleep for 50, 100, 150 or 200 minutes. Some babies will wake and cry demandingly whilst others are content to lie quietly even if they are hungry, wet or a bit uncomfortable, till they drop off again.

In this respect babies are no different from adults. They are all individual, they have different temperaments and different personalities, and these are often apparent almost from the time of birth onwards. One new-born baby may be lying in its crib, arms and legs outstretched, fast asleep with a serene expression on its face, whilst another may come out fighting and lie in its crib, fists clenched, a frown on its forehead, and screaming. It's naive to expect that every baby will behave and sleep like every other baby. Some may just be short sleepers, like adults. Perhaps these are born with an innate curiosity about the world around them, and just simply hate the thought of missing out on anything that's happening in their environment.

If you are the proud but desperate owner of this model, you should not feel that any blame attaches to you. In spite of what many books say, it is very rarely the case that what you do is the cause. In the vast majority of situations parents simply respond to the facts with which they are faced. What they do is an effect of the problem and not its cause.

On the other hand, how you respond under any given set of circumstances can make matters better or worse.

Don't rush in at the first whimper. If you hang on for a few moments you will find that many babies turn over and go back to sleep – how would you like it if every time you grunted, groaned, snorted or shouted out in your sleep, your partner turned on the lights and asked you what was the matter? However, it is not a good idea to wait till your mewling infant has worked itself up to a total paddy – it will take you three times as long to get it back to sleep. Take it a bottle or breast if you think that food is what's needed, keep calm, be reassuring, but above all be confident. Fear of the dark is a very primeval instinct and it may take some little ones much longer to come to terms with feeling comfortable in this situation than others. When you do go, don't turn on the light, but make sure you have a very low watt lamp in the hall or landing and open the baby's door just enough so that you can see what you're doing. Of course, a distressed baby needs love and cuddles but if every time it cries the lights go on, lots of activity happens and it gets lots of attention from its parent, it will very soon learn that this is a smashing trick and you will have been thoroughly conditioned by the baby, just like Pavlov's dogs.

Sometimes the most caring and concerned mothers prolong the agonies for themselves. Several fascinating research studies have shown that children in hospitals or institutions seem to suffer far less disruption of their sleeping patterns. A startling ability of virtually every mother is that of hearing the first peep out of a waking child, regardless of which stage of sleep she's in herself. Even in the depths of the deepest sleep of Stage 4, a mother will be instantly wide awake the moment her child cries, when alarm clocks, telephone bells, the clattering milkman or her snoring partner would all fail to make the slightest impression.

One of the common physical causes which wakes small babies is colic. This usually starts two weeks after birth and affects many babies. Around half of them will be better by their second month but a small percentage are still likely to have problems at four or five months. No one is certain as to the cause of colic, but there does seem to be some link between cow's milk and this unpleasant condition. It occurs more frequently in breastfed babies whose mothers consume a pint (0.5 litre) or more of cow's milk a day. It may also be related to infant feeding formulas, and I have known many mothers successfully overcome this problem by giving up milk themselves or switching their babies to different brands, especially those made up of mainly soya milk.

For centuries dill has been used as a remedy for colic, but many of the modern proprietary brands of gripe water also contain significant amounts of alcohol, which is not a good idea. You can make your own simple remedy from a few crushed dill seeds, a cup of boiling water and a teaspoon of honey. Let it stand for five minutes, strain off the seeds and keep in a tightly stoppered bottle in the fridge until required.

Massage is another sovereign remedy for colic and is most effectively done by putting a towel on your shoulder, lying the baby face down across your shoulder and massaging its back in firm but gentle circular strokes. Some mothers tell me that this works even better if you walk around at the same time.

It's extremely important to establish a familiar, comforting routine for baby's bedtime. Do things in the same order, use the same words, sing the same lullaby. This is not the time to allow Dad in with a new toy or for a tickle, or for a general romp about with the baby, much as they both enjoy it. It's time for peace and quiet. Monotony is a great bringer of sleep, so repetitive movements like rocking, or repetitive sounds are a great aid. There are many 'new age' music cassettes available, and even tapes of heartbeats and whale sounds, and I've had good reports about the use of all of them.

On the subject of music, it's worth considering the whole question of noise. Parents who creep about the house, afraid to turn on the radio or television or talk above a whisper for fear of waking the baby are making a rod for their own back. Just like the person who lives near Heathrow or a railway line gets so used to the noise that they find it difficult to sleep without it, your baby will get used to sleeping in the comforting presence of familiar background domestic sounds. The sooner you start this particular piece of conditioning, the better it will be for all concerned.

Toddlers

From the age of six months onwards there is a gradual reduction in the amount of sleep which the average child needs, so that by the age of two and a half to three most children are likely to be sleeping through the night and having one, or maybe two, naps during the daytime. Unfortunately although sleeping through the night is great, children have a great trick of waking up somewhere around five in the morning. Yet again, individual differences are enormous. Some three-year-olds will happily play, talk to themselves, mutter and wait till they hear stirrings from the rest of the household before making their presence felt. Others will wake at five and want to be up and doing. Unless you want to be up and doing with them, it's best to encourage a certain degree of independence as early as possible, and this raises the whole question of when to swop from cot to bed. I think the only answer to that question is that you make the change when it's no longer safe for the child to sleep in a cot. Once you find your budding Bonnington trying to scale the cot sides, or release the catches that hold it up, he or she is going to be safer in a bed. If they haven't got far to fall they can't do too much damage. At this stage a gate across the staircase is essential (you should have had one as soon as they started to crawl), or even a gate across the bedroom doorway will at least ensure you an extra hour if you're lucky. A bedside light which the child can operate simply and safely, a drink and maybe even a biscuit will help to keep your youngster occupied, together with an easily accessible collection of favourite toys. It's also worth considering a potty in the bedroom if you are in the process of toilet training.

It's important to differentiate between isolated bad nights for which there is an obvious reason, and the persistent non-sleeping child. It's also important to understand that it is not too difficult to turn the former into the latter. Any child that discovers how easy it is to get taken downstairs and cuddled in front of the telly and be given extra drinks and snacks in the middle of the night, just through the simple expedient of having some minor discomfort, is going to have a vested interest in staying awake rather than going to sleep. Wherever possible try to comfort a poorly child in its own bedroom and, as with babies, don't let teething, sore throats, or any other minor ailment become an occasion for family entertainment or play. Quiet music, dim light and the soothing presence of a parent is normally enough. Teething can be a real problem, though certainly it is not the cause of all the illnesses and symptoms for which it gets the blame. One thing is certain, though, and that is that it hurts. Soothing gels, extracts of cloves, even rubbing the gum with an ice cube can all help to assuage this discomfort.

If your child has severe sleeping problems, then it is important to try and solve them as soon as possible. Research at Cardiff University has found that it is more difficult to resolve these irregular sleep patterns after the age of two, and in fact the older the children the longer it took for things to get back to normal. Psychologists have had considerable success using behavioural techniques with these bad sleepers. They used many of the ideas which we've already examined, not making waking periods too enjoyable, not allowing children out of their sleeping environment, and using a mixture of the stick and the carrot. This was done by offering children inducements and rewards for going to bed, things like extra stories if they settled down quickly, special treats if they slept through the night. This type of approach takes time and has to be tackled with calmness, perseverance, resolve and naturally with kindness. It needs to be discussed with the child, and there's no doubt that extra treats are something which any two- or three-year-old understands.

In desperation many parents resort to taking the child into their own bed, and in spite of what all the pundits say, I don't believe there's anything wrong with that as long as you know what you're letting yourself in for. After all, it's only since the Victorian era that children have had separate beds anyway, let along separate rooms, and in many cultures it is normal for whole families to sleep together. It's certainly true that of all the vertebrates, man is the only one that separates babies from their mothers, and then only in what we presume to be civilised societies.

Forget all the myths about suffocating your baby, it doesn't happen. What does happen is that you will probably have to find a different time and place in which to enjoy your sex life, but for some parents if that's the only solution they can find to sleepless nights they consider it a small price to pay. It's important to remember that small children are normally put to bed in babygros, thick pyjamas or warm nighties. Once you bring them into your bed their body temperature will rise considerably, so make sure that you take off their thick night-clothes and put them in something much cooler. Not only will this make sure that they sleep better, but also it's worth noting that there seems to be a link between cot deaths and sudden temperature rises in infants.

Another alternative is to put the child in a separate bed in your room, and again the behavioural approach often works. Once a sleeping routine has been established, try moving the bed further and further away from yours until eventually you're able to put it back into the child's bedroom. Alternatively, try discussing redecoration of the child's room with its would-be occupant, and intimate that once the room is decorated as he or she would like it, it might be a very grown-up thing if the child was to go and sleep in it. What does not work is to have the child in your bed when it suits you, for example during the week when everybody's tired, or when your partner is away for some reason, only to turf the little 'un out again at weekends when you're in the mood for other bedtime activities, or when your partner comes back from his trip. If you've embarked on this course then you have to unravel it slowly and gently.

For some parents a large part of the problem is having sleepless children up and about in what they consider 'their' time. This is a cultural convention which does not exist in other parts of the world. It only needs a holiday in any Mediterranean country to see entire Spanish, Italian or Greek families, toddlers, babes in arms, granny and all strolling to a restaurant at 10 or 11 at night and sitting down to a huge meal. In their society it would be unthinkable to leave the children behind. It is true that the siesta is also part of their tradition, but these late nights have no apparent ill effect whatsoever on the children. Next time you go on holiday, when in Rome . . .

There can be no doubt that children as young as two and upwards suffer stresses and anxieties which affect their sleep, just as they do yours. Imagined fears are just as real – starting school, moving to a new class, worries about their siblings, anxieties about the previous day. It is arrogant and reprehensible to assume that small children are not capable of the same emotional worries as we are.

One family of my patients suffered a tragic cot death when the elder son was five, the mother eight months pregnant and the young brother that died was 19 months. The older child had been very closely attached to his younger brother and was deeply affected by the loss. Having never suffered from any sleep disruption at all, as soon as the new baby arrived he felt compelled to go and look in its cot at almost hourly intervals throughout the night. Understandably this behaviour persisted for several months and it was only by repeatedly talking through his feelings and anxieties that things returned to normal.

If you have established a pattern whereby your child will

only go to sleep with the lights on, try fitting a dimmer switch in the bedroom. This will allow you to reduce the intensity of the light very slightly each two or three days over a period of several weeks. You can do this so slowly that the child hardly notices and eventually you will have a child sleeping in the dark. It's probably a good idea to leave a low watt night-light burning on the landing so that there is a faint glimmer, sufficient to light the way to the bathroom if required.

Nightmares are a constant source of anxiety to parents, but they are a common and perfectly normal function of our dreams. Children's nightmares are no different from adults', nor are the reasons for having them. A child waking with a nightmare will need a lot of comforting and reassuring, but the middle of the night is not the time to try to discuss the content of the dream. Save that for the morning and try to work through the story and uncover the underlying facts behind it if you can.

Night terrors are a different story and it's during this period that they are most likely to happen. They are fairly common but hardly ever continue happening for long, and are much more worrying for the parent than the child. They normally happen during the early part of sleep when the child will sit bolt upright in bed, eyes staring and screaming in abject terror. The effect on parents when it happens for the first time is appalling, but be reassured that there is nothing to be alarmed about. The child will be inconsolable and all you can do is to hug and comfort the wretched infant, who will eventually go back to sleep and remember nothing the following morning. Night terrors are most likely at times of stress, so it is important to try to sort out the root of the problem. Again it's useless to do this in the middle of the night, but don't avoid doing it the following day.

Sleep-walking can be quite a serious problem in children in so far as they can come to harm. If you have a sleep-walker make sure that you take all the practical precautions you can to avoid accidents. Like night terrors they seem to be stress-related and to run in families. A lot of children who start with night terrors progress to sleep-walking, but it rarely persists into adolescence or adulthood.

One particular habit which is often overlooked as a cause of disturbed sleep is tooth-grinding or bruxism. This happens during sleep when the jaws are clenched and the teeth ground together. Most tooth-grinding children are unaware of what they are doing but can be woken up by pain in the temporomandibular joints. Those are the big joints just in front of the ears where the lower jaw hinges into the upper jaw. Not only does this strange habit disturb the sleep, it can also do considerable damage to the teeth, wearing away the enamel, causing uneven wear and subsequent stress on the joints of the jaw. The muscle tension produced by these uneven stresses can lead to recurrent headaches or even migraine. Tooth-grinding is a specific sign of underlying tension and anxiety. Your dentist can help by making adjustments to the child's bite, or by fitting a specially made bite guard, but these will only help the symptoms; you will need to find the cause of your child's anxiety.

Hyperactivity

In recent years there has been much controversy surrounding the question of hyperactive children. This term does not apply to those who are simply naughty or badly behaved, or even difficult. It applies to children who are impossible. They are disruptive, destructive both to themselves and to property, they can be violent and extremely aggressive, they have short attention spans and great difficulty in concentrating, they have learning difficulties, they never sit still and they don't sleep.

For years these children were treated exclusively as behaviourally disturbed until, in the late '60s, Dr Ben Feingold, an allergist working in America, stumbled across a possible chemical cause for hyperactivity quite by accident. Whilst working on a project connected to flea-bite allergies in children, he devised a special diet which excluded a group of chemicals called salicylates – related to the aspirin family and similar to the substances produced by fleas. A number of children who were extremely allergic to flea bites were put on this diet and Feingold was astounded when many of the parents told him that not only were the children reacting less severely to the flea bites, but their behaviour had improved as well.

He then began a large-scale study on hyperactive children

who had been institutionalised as they were beyond control. A considerable percentage of the children responded dramatically to the diet, their behaviour changing within days. When they were challenged with a doughnut filled with artificially coloured and flavoured jam, their behaviour deteriorated within hours. What Feingold had established was that many of the chemicals used as artificial food additives were salicylates, and he suggested that it was these very chemicals together with natural salicylates occurring in some foods, that were the root of the problem for some children.

If your sleepless child also shows signs of hyperactivity, it is certainly worth trying Feingold's diet for three or four weeks. Even non-hyperactive children who are non-sleepers may be sensitive to some of the chemicals. Amongst the worst offenders is the yellow colouring tartrazine, E102, which is widespread in convenience foods and especially in many of the drinks, sweets and biscuits aimed directly at the children's market. Over the last 20 years I've seen dozens of children (and their parents) restored to sleep by the simple expedient of avoiding food additives. It's worth noting that some of these can also be the trigger for asthmatic attacks, eczema, urticaria and other itches and irritations.

The Allergy Diet

This diet is based on the original work of Dr Ben Feingold. For the past 20 years I have been applying his theories to the practical problems of dealing with hyperactive, asthmatic, allergic and even, in some instances, epileptic children. I don't promise that it will solve your child's sleep problems, but unlike some extreme exclusion diets it cannot do any harm, and will inevitably be healthier than most youngsters' normal eating habits. Eliminating all the chemicals can only be beneficial and you may be one of the lucky families for whom this diet does the trick. The instructions for following the diet may seem onerous to start with but there has been a gratifying improvement in the range of additive-free foods now in the marketplace. You will probably find a wide selection in any health food store, but you will also be able to purchase a huge variety of suitable foods in your local supermarket.

Persevere. It's no good going off half-cock as you will not achieve any degree of success unless you do it properly as follows:-

1. Keep a diet diary and write down *everything* your child eats. It's important to keep this diary going even after any improvements have occurred. If there is a sudden return to the old hyperactive behaviour, the diary will provide a record so that you can check on any lapses that may have occurred. These should be rare if the diet is carefully monitored, but if there has been a slip and some forbidden food has been consumed, behavioural changes can happen as quickly as two hours later.

It's worth keeping a column in the diary for general behaviour and school progress. If the diet is working but there is any sudden deterioration in behaviour, suspect that one or other of the baddies has crept in, either by accident or by stealth on the part of your child.

2. Any fruit or vegetable which is not on the prohibitied list of Group I is allowed. Sometimes a child may have its own individual allergy or adverse reaction to any food. If you suspect this then add that food to the forbidden list.

3. You have to become a dedicated label reader and reject any product which you are not certain is free of artificial additives. If a product doesn't describe colours or flavours as natural, don't buy it. If you can't be 100% sure, it's not worth experimenting.

4. Nearly all the permitted foods are available off the supermarket shelf and you should not have to pay a hefty premium just to avoid the chemicals.

5. All children enjoy the occasional sweet and it is not reasonable to ban these totally from the diet. Unfortunately virtually all commercial confectionery contains the suspect chemicals, so in order to avoid them and still allow your child treats, you will have to make at home things like cakes, biscuits, pies, pastries, puddings and even simple sweets. There are many recipe books which will tell you how to do this.

Ice cream is another favourite which it is difficult to obtain commercially without additives. Even if the ice cream itself is prepared without them, the fruits, nuts or chocolate which they contain are probably not.

6. The best way to ensure success is to get the whole family following the diet. This is not as hard as it sounds, the list provides a very varied and liberal selection of foods and not having any of the prohibited items in the house does remove temptation and the risk of infringements. It is also very unfair to expect young children not to feel persecuted if they are forbidden certain foods when their brothers and sisters, or for that matter their parents, sit in front of them eating all the goodies which they're not allowed.

The initial restriction on fresh fruits and the two vegetables does not normally need to be continued for very long. If there are obvious benefits from the diet it is normally in order to start reintroducing them after four to six weeks. Only give one new food in any 48-hour period so that you can spot those that might still present a problem.

If the hyperactive child sees the entire family willing to make sacrifices in order to help, then the incentive for the child to stick to the regime will be considerably reinforced.

7. If you are going to succeed, this must be a 100% effort. 80%, 90% or even 95% will not work. For some children one bite of a food containing the suspect chemicals is enough to trigger an adverse response and this may continue for 72 hours or more. If your child has a mouthful of tartrazine on Sunday, and another on Wednesday, it could keep him or her in a hyperactive state for a whole week.

8. Usually a good response will be obvious within seven to 21 days; in some children behavioural improvements may be noticed within two or three days of changing the diet, in others it might take seven weeks. If your child is one of those sensitive to, or allergic to, these chemicals then you will see a benefit for all your efforts, so persevere.

9. Severely hyperactive children are frequently prescribed behaviour-modifying drugs and you should never make changes to your child's medication without consulting the family doctor. It is very rewarding to watch your child improve and manage on reduced doses of drugs and frequently, when these dietary changes do have a positive effect, medication can

be stopped altogether after three to four weeks. This is true even after months or years of medication. If the child has been on tranquillising drugs the withdrawal effects can be quite dramatic and the period for coming off can stretch to two or three months. This too must not be attempted without involving your GP (see page 78).

Until recently many of the drugs prepared for children contained some of the very chemicals as flavourings and colourings which we now know cause problems in some children. Many pediatric preparations are now available without additives, so check with your doctor or pharmacist to make sure you get these for your child.

It sometimes happens that after starting the diet, behaviour-modifying drugs can have a stimulating rather than sedative effect. If your child shows this type of response consult your doctor.

All this may look formidable but not half so formidable as trying to cope with a hyperactive insomniac. Please remember that this diet is not a universal panacea for all children with behavioural problems. For the percentage of children who are sensitive to the salicylate and other chemical additives it can work like a dream.

Two groups of food are eliminated by the diet:

Group I is made up of a number of fruits and two vegetables (tomato and cucumber). This group of foods contains natural salicylates.

Group II is made up of all foods that contain a synthetic (artificial) colour or flavour.

There are no tests to determine whether a child will show an unfavourable behavioural response to any food item in either Group I or II. The allergy skin tests for foods are not applicable to this problem.

In the absence of tests it is necessary to start the diet by eliminating *every* food that might disturb the child from Group I and those foods not permitted in Group II.

Group I

This is the list of fruits and vegetables that contain natural salicylates. They must be omitted in any and all forms – fresh, frozen, canned, dried, as juice or as an ingredient of prepared foods.

Fruits

Almonds

Apples
Apricots
Berries:
  Blackberries
  Gooseberries
  Raspberries
  Strawberries
Cherries
Currants
Grapes and raisins or any product made of grapes, e.g. wine, wine vinegar, jellies, etc.
Nectarines
Oranges (Note: grapefruit, lemon and lime are permitted)
Peaches
Plums and prunes

Vegetables

Tomatoes and all tomato products
Cucumbers (pickles)

If the child shows a favourable response to the diet, after four to six weeks the foods in Group I may be slowly restored. The intolerance to these foods is usually related to aspirin-sensitivity. Since aspirin-sensitivity in children is often difficult to detect, a history of such intolerance in the parents is used as a guide. If one or the other parent offers a history of aspirin-sensitivity, caution must be exercised in reintroducing the fruits and vegetables in Group I.

Try the foods *one at a time* for about three or four days. If no unfavourable reaction in the child's behaviour is noted, another item can be added. This procedure is followed until all items in Group I are tested and those to which there is no adverse reaction are restored to the diet.

Group II

All foods that contain artificial colour and artificial flavour are prohibited. The following list is meant to serve as a guide for shopping and food preparation.

It should be emphasised that this diet is not concerned with food preservatives except for Butylated Hydroxy Toluene (BHT). An occasional child may show an adverse response to BHT.

All foods that contain artificial colour and artificial flavours are not listed. Such a list is not practical. Do not use *any* foods that contain these substances.

The safest approach is to read the labels carefully. Upon checking in the market, a number of items will be found to contain *no* artificial colour or flavour.

There are some permitted food items that must be prepared at home to avoid synthetics.

From present indications, an individual sensitive to artificial colours and flavours must avoid them throughout his life.

Not Permitted	**Permitted**
Cereals	*Cereals*
All cereals with artificial colours and flavours	Any cereal without artificial colours or flavours, dry or cooked
All instant-breakfast preparations	
Bakery Goods	*Bakery Goods*
All manufactured cakes, pastries, sweet rolls, doughnuts, etc. Pie crusts	Any product without artificial colour or flavour, but most bakery items must be prepared at home
Frozen baked goods	

Foods to avoid	Permitted foods
Many packaged baking mixes	All commercial breads except egg bread and whole wheat (usually dyed, unless 100% wholewheat, e.g. Allinsons)
Luncheon Meats Bologna Salami Frankfurters Sausages* Meat loaf Ham, bacon, pork *(When coloured or flavoured, usually indicated on the package)	*All Meats*
Poultry All barbecued types All turkeys with prepared basting called 'self-basting', prepared stuffing	*All Poultry except Stuffed*
Fish Frozen fish fillets that are dyed or flavoured; fish sticks that are dyed or flavoured	*All Fresh Fish*
Desserts Manufactured ice creams, unless the label specifies no synthetic colouring or flavouring; the same applies to sherbet, ices, gelatines, junkets, puddings All powdered puddings All dessert mixes	*Desserts* Homemade ice cream without artificial colouring or flavouring Gelatines – homemade from pure gelatines, with any permitted natural fruit or fruit juices Tapioca Homemade custards and puddings

Flavoured yoghurt

Plain yoghurt – permitted fresh fruits or juice may be added

Sweets

All manufactured types, hard or soft

Sweets

Homemade sweets without almonds

Beverages

Cider
Wine
Beer
Diet juices
Soft drinks
All instant breakfast drinks
All quick-mix powdered drinks
Tea, hot or cold
Prepared chocolate milk
Coffee

Beverages

Grapefruit juice
Pineapple juice
Pear nectar
Guava nectar
Homemade lemonade or limeade from fresh lemons or limes
Milk

Miscellaneous Items

Any margarine containing artificial additives
Coloured butter
Mustard
All mint-flavoured items
Soy sauce if flavoured or coloured
Cider vinegar
Wine vinegar
Commercial chocolate syrup
Barbecue-flavoured potato chips
Cloves
Ketchup
Chilli sauce
Coloured cheeses

Miscellaneous Items

All cooking oils and fats

Butter icing, not coloured or flavoured
Mustard prepared at home from pure powder and distilled vinegar
Jams or jellies made from permitted fruits, not artificially coloured or flavoured
Honey
Homemade mayonnaise
Distilled white vinegar
Homemade chocolate syrup for all purposes
All natural (white) cheeses

Sundry Items

Many pediatric medicines and vitamins contain artificial colour and flavour as well as sugar. If your child needs any medication do ask advice from your doctor or pharmacist.

A lot of over-the-counter medications contain aspirin, as well as artificial flavours and colours. Be particularly careful of pain-killers, cold cures, cough remedies and anti-histamines.

All toothpastes and toothpower
(A salt-and-soda mixture
can be used for cleaning
teeth. Neutrogena soap –
unscented – can be
substituted for toothpaste
or powder.)
All mouthwashes
All cough drops
All throat lozenges
Antacid tablets
Perfumes

Other Childhood Complaints

Lice and worms can also be chronic destroyers of your child's sleep, and yours. Contrary to popular mythology, lice have nothing to do with dirt, the fact is that the favourite habitat of the louse is short, clean hair. You can't catch lice from somebody else's comb, hat, hairbrush, off the mat in the school gym or off the back of the bus seat. Lice can only be transferred from head to head by direct physical contact. Louse shampoos are, on the whole, not much use – all you get is clean lice. The special applications which you leave on the head for a decent period of time are more effective, but the most effective deterrent of all is a comb. This does not need to be the fine-toothed nit comb which is difficult and painful to use, but any good quality, reasonably fine comb will do. Lice cling to the hair with their legs. When you dislodge them from the hair you break off a leg or two and a legless louse is a dead louse! It's also worth remembering that the louse is a classless creature, it has no preference and will happily reside on the head of anyone's child.

Sadly the disappearance of the louse nurse from our school system has meant a revival of its fortunes, and an infestation of headlice makes children feel 'lousy'. The itching and scratching will keep your child awake as sure as lice have nits.

Any child that claims it can't get to sleep because of an itchy bottom may well be suffering from threadworms. These unpleasant little creatures have a nasty and inconvenient habit of deciding to wriggle out through your child's anus just when it's time to go to bed. Any visible signs of these fine, threadlike creatures should result in a quick visit to your GP.

There are several practical considerations which will help to make life easier for all of you. No child will sleep well in an uncomfortable lumpy bed, or with a knobbly compressed baby's pillow which has been handed down for the fourth time. It might seem like obvious common sense, but your baby or small child can't tell you when it's uncomfortable, so do look at the mattress and pillow carefully.

Herb pillows can be extremely effective in helping your child to sleep (see page 102). Cold, hunger, indigestion, wind and a full bladder do nothing to help. Make sure the room is warm enough, but not too warm, that your child has been fed, but not too late, and that its bladder is empty. It's sometimes worth waking a child just before you go to bed and taking it to the toilet. This also helps with simple bedwetting problems.

Sugar and children are not a healthy mixture at any time, but it does seem as though sweetened drinks or sugary snacks late at night can interfere with sleep. Milk is a natural source of tryptophan (see page 76), which is probably the reason that warm milky drinks, especially those which contain some carbohydrate like Horlicks, seem to work.

I am frequently disturbed by the ease with which many doctors write prescriptions for powerful drugs intended for sleepless children. It is true that matters can sometimes get to breaking point, but tranquillisers and hypnotics should be absolutely the last resort. All these drugs can have side effects and can be addictive (see Chapter 5). I sympathise with the desperate parents of insomniac children, but you must avoid the temptation to dose them with over-the-counter medicines which have sedative actions. Many cough medicines, pain killers and anti-histamines can be used in this way and frequently are. Even more hazardous is giving small children medicaments prescribed for adults, as the body weight to dose ratio can result in very large overdoses.

Try some of the simple herbal remedies like chamomile tea sweetened with a little honey (see page 90), or any of the homeopathic preparations which are cheap, absolutely safe and often extremely effective. It is surely worth consulting a homeopathic physician who will look not just at the child but at the whole environment in which it is living, including you.

It is never too early to use some of the relaxation techniques (see page 122). Small babies, toddlers and adolescents will all enjoy some relaxing and soothing massage and it is possible to teach even very young children the rudiments of relaxation exercises and simple yoga.

Finally a word of consolation. There is no evidence that children who don't sleep are necessarily very bright, or that children who sleep a lot are necessarily less bright. What is true is that many gifted children are very poor sleepers, and for this special minority additional mental stimulus is often the trick that turns the tide and gets them off to sleep.

I believe that lack of physical activity and mental boredom can play a part in a large percentage of children's sleep disorders. Keep your children both physically and mentally occupied, stretch them and encourage them to use their minds and bodies. Don't go too far because the overtired child, like the overtired adult, will have difficulties in getting to sleep.

ENDPIECE

THE EMERGENCY SURVIVAL GUIDE TO INSOMNIA

'Sleep is when all the unsorted stuff comes flying out as from a dustbin upset in a high wind.'

Wiliam Golding

Whether you are a chronic insomniac who has finally decided to do something about it or you are just suffering the disturbing experience of your first ever episode of this distressing condition, here are some simple steps which will help you on the road to the peace and sense of well-being that a good night's sleep brings.

First, you must determine that the solution to your problems lies largely in your own mind and your own hands. It's no good relying on others to solve the problem for you, and it's even worse to struggle through life on the crutch of drug or alcohol dependency. Whatever you do, don't panic. No-one can stay awake forever, and when you are sufficiently tired you will sleep. Everyone who has a sleep problem has a very false idea of how much or how little they sleep. The perception of sleep is very different from the reality, and all sleep laboratory experiments have shown that insomniacs sleep for far longer than they believe they do.

Here is a summary of some of the simple things which are most likely to help you.

1. Ignore all old wives' tales. You will not go mad if you don't dream, you will grow if you don't sleep, one hour's sleep at any time of the night is worth one hour's sleep.

2. Regulate your own time clock. No matter what time you go to bed, you must get up at the same time each morning.

3. There is no such thing as a 'normal' amount of sleep. You need whatever you need – that may be quite different from what your parents, wife, mother-in-law or next door neighbour needs. If you do have a few nights of less sleep than you like, don't worry – nothing terrible is going to happen to you except that you will feel more tired in the daytime.

4. If you smoke, give it up, or at least try to do without cigarettes late at night – and never smoke in bed.

5. Drastically reduce your intake of caffeine in coffee, tea, chocolate and cola drinks. There are now caffeine-free substitutes available everywhere.

6. Don't go to bed hungry, and don't go to bed on a stomach full of heavy, greasy, indigestible food.

7. Make sure that the temperature of your bedroom is suitable – not too hot and not too cold. Somewhere between 60–70°F (15–21°C) seems comfortable for most people.

8. Look to your bed, your bedclothes and your night clothes. Most people change their cars every two or three years, their television every five or six and their fridge and washing machine every six to eight. Beds, on the other hand, are expected to last a lifetime. They don't. Is your bedding the way you would like it? Is it too heavy or too light? Too warm or too cold? Experiment until you find the best solution. Does your pyjama cord tangle up round your middle? Does your nightie end up round your neck? Perhaps you'd be better off sleeping in the nude.

9. Never use alcohol to help you get to sleep.

10. Never go on crash diets or take any form of slimming pills unless prescribed by your own, regular, family doctor.

11. A slight rise in body temperature helps you get to sleep, so a 15-minute soak in a warm bath, using some of the relaxing herbal extracts (see page 93) is a great aid.

12. Learn to cope with the stresses and strains of your daily life by taking up any of the relaxation techniques (see page 122).

13. Try to control your body weight. Don't let it go up or down too much. And stick to regular mealtimes. This is particularly important in the evening.

14. Take up some form of regular exercise. It doesn't matter what, as long as it's appropriate to your age and physical condition. What does matter is regularity. Aim for half an hour each day of anything which makes you get out of breath.

15. Don't ruminate. Going over and over yesterday's, last week's or last year's battles with the boss or family feuds is a certain recipe for insomnia. There is no point in worrying about things you can't change. Try to endure these with strength. Have the courage to tackle things you can change and the wisdom to know the difference.

16. Finally, if you get to that point in the night when repose is tabooed by anxiety, your bedclothes are in a tangle and your pillow steadfastly refuses to stay where it makes you comfortable, get up, do something which is not over-stimulating, don't have a cup of tea or coffee – any other warm drink may help – and don't go back to bed until you feel sleepy. Which you will – I promise. No matter what time this happens, leave your alarm clock set for its normal hour – even if you don't have to get up.

Insomnia is not a disease, it's a condition which your body has got into by default. You can do something about it providing you have the will and the determination. But whatever you do – don't just lie there!

INDEX